Pediatric Sleep Clinics

Editor

HAVIVA VELER

SLEEP MEDICINE CLINICS

www.sleep.theclinics.com

June 2023 • Volume 18 • Number 2

ELSEVIER

1600 John F. Kennedy Boulevard • Suite 1800 • Philadelphia, Pennsylvania, 19103-2899

http://www.theclinics.com

SLEEP MEDICINE CLINICS Volume 18, Number 2
June 2023, ISSN 1556-407X, ISBN-13: 978-0-323-94003-0

Editor: Joanna Collett
Developmental Editor: Axell Ivan Jade M. Purificacion

Sleep Medicine Clinics (ISSN 1556-407X) is published quarterly by Elsevier Inc., 360 Park Avenue South, New York, NY 10010-1710. Months of issue are March, June, September and December. Business and Editorial Offices: 1600 John F. Kennedy Blvd., Ste. 1800, Philadelphia, PA 19103-2899. Customer Service Office: 3251 Riverport Lane, Maryland Heights, MO 63043. Periodicals postage paid at New York, NY and additional mailing offices. Subscription prices are $243.00 per year (US individuals), $100.00 (US and Canadian students), $612.00 (US institutions), $283.00 (Canadian individuals), $278.00 (international individuals) $135.00 (International students), $692.00 (Canadian and International institutions). Foreign air speed delivery is included in all *Clinics* subscription prices. All prices are subject to change without notice. **POSTMASTER:** Send change of address to *Sleep Medicine Clinics*, Elsevier Health Sciences Division, Subscription Customer Service, 3251 Riverport Lane, Maryland Heights, MO 63043. Customer Service: **Tel: 1-800-654-2452 (U.S. and Canada); 314-447-8871 (outside U.S. and Canada). Fax: 314-447-8029. E-mail: journalscustomerservice-usa@elsevier.com (for print support); journalsonline-support-usa@elsevier.com (for online support).**

Reprints. For copies of 100 or more of articles in this publication, please contact the Commercial Reprints Department, Elsevier Inc., 360 Park Avenue South, New York, NY 10010-1710. Tel.: 212-633-3874; Fax: 212-633-3820; E-mail: reprints@elsevier.com.

Sleep Medicine Clinics is covered in *MEDLINE/PubMed (Index Medicus)*.

SLEEP MEDICINE CLINICS

SERIES OF RELATED INTEREST

Psychiatric Clinics
https://www.psych.theclinics.com/

THE CLINICS ARE AVAILABLE ONLINE!
Access your subscription at:
www.theclinics.com

Contributors

CONSULTING EDITORS

TEOFILO LEE-CHIONG Jr, MD
Professor of Medicine, National Jewish Health,
Professor of Medicine, University of Colorado,
Denver, Colorado, USA; Chief Medical Liaison,
Philips Respironics, Murrysville, Pennsylvania,
USA

ANA C. KRIEGER, MD, MPH, FCCP, FAASM
Chief, Division of Sleep Neurology, Medical
Director, Weill Cornell Center for Sleep
Medicine, Professor of Clinical Medicine,
Professor of Medicine in Neurology and
Genetic Medicine, Weill Cornell Medical
College, Cornell University, New York, New
York, USA

EDITOR

HAVIVA VELER, MD, FAASM
Head, Division of Pediatric Pulmonology and
Sleep Medicine, Connecticut Children's Medical
Center, Associate Professor, University of
Connecticut, University of Connecticut School of
Medicine, Hartford, Connecticut, USA

AUTHORS

BAHA AL-SHAWWA, MD
Division of Pulmonary and Sleep Medicine,
Children's Mercy Hospital, Kansas City,
Missouri, USA

JULIE M. BAUGHN, MD
Division of Pulmonary and Critical Care, Mayo
Clinic Center for Sleep Medicine, Mayo Clinic,
Rochester, Minnesota, USA

MARGARET BLATTNER, MD, PhD
Instructor, Department of Neurology, Beth
Israel Deaconess Medical Center, Harvard
Medical School, Boston, Massachusetts, USA

OLIVIERO BRUNI, MD
Department of Social and Developmental
Psychology, Sapienza University, Rome, Italy

CORINNE CATAROZOLI, PhD
Assistant Professor of Psychology in Clinical
Psychiatry, Assistant Professor of Psychology
in Clinical Pediatrics, Department of
Psychiatry, Weill Cornell Medicine, New York,
New York, USA

CHRISTOPHER M. CIELO, DO, MSTR
Assistant Professor of Pediatrics, Division
of Pulmonary and Sleep Medicine,
Children's Hospital of Philadelphia,
Perelman School of Medicine, University of
Pennsylvania, Philadelphia, Pennsylvania,
USA

TAMIKA A. CRANFORD, MHPE, RRT-NPS, RPSGT, CCSH
Division of Pulmonary and Sleep Medicine,
Children's Mercy Hospital, Kansas City,
Missouri, USA

LOURDES M. DELROSSO, MD, PhD
University of California, San Francisco,
University Sleep and Pulmonary Associates,
Fresno, California, USA

RAFFAELE FERRI, MD
Department of Neurology I.C., Sleep Research
Centre, Oasi Research Institute - IRCCS,
Troina, Italy

ALICE M. GREGORY, PhD
Department of Psychology, Goldsmiths, University of London, London, United Kingdom

DAVID G. INGRAM, MD, MHPE
Division of Pulmonary and Sleep Medicine, Children's Mercy Hospital, Kansas City, Missouri, USA

SHERYL JOHNSON, MD
Clinical Resident, Division of Pediatrics, Children Hospital of New Jersey at Newark Beth Israel Hospital, Newark, New Jersey, USA

MICHAL KAHN, PhD
School of Psychological Sciences, Tel Aviv University, Tel Aviv, Israel; College of Education, Psychology and Social Work, Flinders University, Bedford Park, South Australia, Australia

ELIOT S. KATZ, MD
Assistant Professor, Division of Respiratory Diseases, Boston Children's Hospital, Harvard Medical School, Boston, Massachusetts, USA

FRANCESCA LUPINI, MS
Clinical Research Coordinator, Children's National Hospital, Washington, DC, USA

KIRAN MASKI, MD, MPH
Associate Professor, Department of Neurology, Boston Children's Hospital, Harvard Medical School, Boston, Massachusetts, USA

CHRISTINE A. MATARESE, DO
Division of Pulmonary and Critical Care, Mayo Clinic Center for Sleep Medicine, Mayo Clinic, Rochester, Minnesota, USA

LISA J. MELTZER, PhD
National Jewish Health, University of Colorado Denver, Anschutz Medical Campus, Denver, Colorado, USA

MARIA PAOLA MOGAVERO, MD
Institute of Molecular Bioimaging and Physiology, National Research Council, Division of Neuroscience, Sleep Disorders Center, San Raffaele Scientific Institute, Centro di Medicina Del Sonno, IRCCS Ospedale San Raffaele, Milano, Italy

ISABEL MORALES-MUÑOZ, PhD
Institute for Mental Health, School of Psychology, University of Birmingham, Birmingham, United Kingdom

COURTNEY PAISLEY, PhD
University of Colorado Denver, Anschutz Medical Campus, Children's Hospital Colorado, Developmental Pediatrics, Aurora, Colorado, USA

IGNACIO E. TAPIA, MD, MSTR
Associate Professor of Pediatrics, Division of Pulmonary and Sleep Medicine, Children's Hospital of Philadelphia, Perelman School of Medicine, University of Pennsylvania, Philadelphia, Pennsylvania, USA

HAVIVA VELER, MD, FAASM
Head, Division of Pediatric Pulmonology and Sleep Medicine, Connecticut Children's Medical Center, Associate Professor, University of Connecticut, University of Connecticut School of Medicine, Hartford, Connecticut, USA

ARIEL A. WILLIAMSON, PhD, DBSM
Assistant Professor and Licensed Psychologist, Children's Hospital of Philadelphia, Roberts Center for Pediatric Research, University of Pennsylvania, Perelman School of Medicine, Philadelphia, Pennsylvania, USA

STEPHANIE O. ZANDIEH, MD, MS
Clinical Assistant Professor, Division Director of Pediatric Pulmonary and Sleep Medicine, Division of Pediatrics, Cooperman Barnabas Medical Center, Children Hospital of New Jersey at Newark Beth Israel Hospital, New Jersey Medical School, West Orange, New Jersey, USA

Contents

> Obstructive sleep apnea (OSA) is common children. There is a demand for more family-focused evaluation and novel diagnostic approaches. Drug-induced sleep endoscopy is increasingly being used clinically in children with Down syndrome and other comorbidities. Several studies have examined the association between OSA and other comorbidities during childhood. Therapeutic options for OSA in children remain limited. Recent studies have examined the utility of hypoglossal nerve stimulation in children with Down syndrome. Positive airway pressure has been a mainstay of OSA treatment. Several recent studies have assessed factors associated with adherence. Infants are challenging to treat for OSA.

> Narcolepsy types 1 and 2 and idiopathic hypersomnia are primary Central Nervous System (CNS) disorders of hypersomnolence characterized by profound daytime sleepiness and/or excessive sleep need. Onset of symptoms begins typically in childhood or adolescence, and children can have unique presentations compared with adults. Narcolepsy type 1 is likely caused by immune-mediated loss of orexin (hypocretin) neurons in the hypothalamus; however, the causes of narcolepsy type 2 and idiopathic hypersomnia are unknown. Existing treatments improve daytime sleepiness and cataplexy but there is no cure for these disorders.

> Restless legs syndrome (RLS) affects 2% of children presenting with symptoms of insomnia, restless sleep, decreased quality of life, and effects on cognition and behavior. The International RLS Study Group and the American Academy of Sleep Medicine have published guidelines for the diagnosis and treatment of RLS in children. Restless sleep disorder has been recently identified in children and presents with frequent movements during sleep and daytime symptoms with polysomnography findings of at least 5 large muscle movements at night. Treatment options for both disorders include iron supplementation, either oral or intravenous with improvement in nighttime and daytime symptoms.

> Sleep and inflammatory cytokines have a bidirectional relationship where circadian rhythms influence increase in levels of certain cytokines, and in return, some cytokines induce sleep, as we frequently experience during illnesses. The most commonly studied cytokines, in the context of inflammation and sleep, are interleukin 6 (IL-6), tumor necrosis factor (TNF), and (IL-1). In this article, the author follows the effect of circadian rhythms on blood levels of these cytokines and explores the changes in their levels in conditions that affect sleep, such as obstructive sleep apnea and insomnia.

> The coronavirus disease 2019 (COVID-19) pandemic has significantly affected childhood sleep. Decreased sleep quality and duration, more bedtime resistance, difficulty initiating and maintaining sleep, and higher rates of parasomnias have all

been noted. The mental health crisis with doubling rates of anxiety and depression has also had a profound influence on youth sleep. The pediatric sleep medicine field has responded to the COVID-19 pandemic by adapting existing practices for safety and greatly expanding telemedicine services. Research and training considerations are further discussed.

This article reviews disparities in pediatric sleep health and sleep disorders from early childhood through adolescence (birth to age 18 years). Sleep health is a multi-dimensional construct including sleep duration, consolidation, and other domains, whereas sleep disorders reflect both behaviorally (eg, insomnia) and medically based (eg, sleep disordered breathing) sleep diagnoses. Using a socioecological framework, we review multilevel (ie, child, family, school, health-care system, neighborhood, and sociocultural) factors linked to sleep health disparities. Mechanistic research and studies using an intersectional lens to understand overlapping marginalized identities are needed to inform multilevel interventions to promote sleep health equity in pediatrics.

Pediatric sleep providers frequently encounter issues related to sleep technology in clinical settings. In this review article, we discuss technical issues related to standard polysomnography, research on putative complementary novel metrics derived from polysomnographic signals as well as research on home sleep apnea testing in children and consumer sleep devices. Although developments across several of these domains are exciting, it remains a rapidly evolving area. When evaluating innovative devices and home sleep testing approaches, clinicians should be mindful of accurately interpreting diagnostic agreement statistics to apply these technologies appropriately.

Previous reviews have described the links between sleep and mental health extensively. In this narrative review, we focus on literature published during the last decade investigating the links between sleep and mental health difficulties in childhood and adolescence. More specifically, we focus on the mental health disorders listed in the most recent edition of the Diagnostic and Statistical Manual of Mental Disorders. We also discuss possible mechanisms underlying these associations. The review ends with a discussion of possible future lines of enquiry.

Preface
Pediatric Sleep Health and Illnesses: An Update

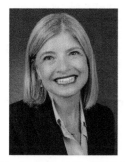

Haviva Veler, MD, FAASM
Editor

The concept that pediatric sleep health and issues are distinctly different compared with sleep medicine as it is known in adults was initially presented in the 1970s. Since then, a fascinating journey of discovery took place, from the description of fundamentals of normal sleep in the different ages, through defining and creating treatment plans to a variety of sleep issues. Recently, a new concept was brought up, describing sleep as a pillar of health and normal development rather than as an illness, and as such, should have a forefront place in discussions of wellness in children's well visits and in parent's conversations.

In this issue, the wide range of topics covered, the wealth of information included, and the quality of research encompassed not only provide compelling evidence for how far we have come but also offer a template for future clinical and research directions.

This issue starts with elaborate description of normal sleep through the ages. The recognition that normal sleep has future implications on a child's growth, development, and future achievements places a great weight on monitoring, maintaining, and advocating for normal sleep. In addition, having a framework for normal sleep, as published by the American Academy of Pediatrics in 2016, provides

a base for recommendations. Because sleep is a pillar of health, rather than a pathologic condition, knowing how to evaluate and maintain good sleep requires guidelines for parents and primary providers, a topic that is discussed.

We continue with looking at insomnia through the ages, checking causes and treatment options, as well as looking at circadian rhythm disorders, commonly seen in adolescents and requiring attention by parents, providers, and specialists. An exploration of the diagnosis and treatments is available for restless leg syndrome, as well as the newly described restless sleep disorder that is unique in pediatrics.

Highlights and new findings in sleep topics are reviewed. After delving into sleep issues in pediatrics, an overview of obstructive sleep apnea provides an up-to-date review of new approaches to this complex and constantly developing field. A look at special populations commonly affected by the condition provides newly available treatment options.

The hypersomnia syndromes are discussed with a specific look at new findings in the field of narcolepsy.

New and recent developments in pediatric sleep, such as the effects of the SARS-CoV-2

Sleep Med Clin 18 (2023) xi–xii
https://doi.org/10.1016/j.jsmc.2023.03.001

pandemic on children's sleep, are discussed. The important topic of sleep as a reflection of health disparities and the differences in concepts and beliefs of normal sleep among different populations takes a forefront seat.

Sleep can be addressed and discussed when a reliable measurement is available, and we dive into the new world of consumer products to review availability of monitors and their validation.

By combining updated reviews on sleep problems, reviewing and addressing sleep as a health maintenance and not an illness, as well as by looking into newly emerging topics in pediatric sleep, we hope to bring you a vibrant and most updated review of pediatric sleep.

Haviva Veler, MD, FAASM
Division of Pediatric Pulmonology and
Sleep Medicine
Connecticut Children's Medical Center
University of Connecticut
85 Seymour Street
Suite 500
Hartford, CT 06106, USA

E-mail address:
hveler@connecticutchildrens.org

Sleep from Infancy Through Adolescence

Stephanie O. Zandieh, MD, MS[a], Sheryl Johnson, MD[b], Eliot S. Katz, MD[c],*

KEYWORDS

- Sleep • Infant • Toddler • School-aged children • Adolescents • Sleep duration • Sleep timing
- Sleep efficiency

KEY POINTS

- Pediatric sleep is characterized by considerable interindividual and night-to-night variability in sleep timing and duration.
- The structure of sleep in infants and children evolves over time, with longer sleep duration, shorter sleep cycles, and more rapid eye movement sleep in infants, and a delayed circadian phase and less slow-wave sleep in adolescence.
- Infants have a more collapsible upper airway and lower lung volumes than older children, which predisposes them to obstructive sleep apnea and sleep-related hypoxemia.

INTRODUCTION

Sleep is a universal need and an active process that changes dramatically from infancy through adolescence. Sleep-wake patterns are distinguished through a constellation of behavioral and physiologic changes. The following characteristics establish sleep from wakefulness: (1) behavioral quiescence when motor activity may be reduced; (2) adoption of specific postures; (3) elevated arousal thresholds so that a higher-intensity stimulus is required to elicit a response; (4) rapid, spontaneous reversibility; (5) homeostatic regulation, which drives sleep in response to sleep deprivation; and (6) partial governance by circadian or ultradian biorhythms.[1] Sleep has an age-specific timing, duration, state distribution, electroencephalogram (EEG) microarchitecture, and respiratory physiology, which are reviewed.

Defining what constitutes "normal" or "optimal" sleep for any age range is difficult because sleep has many dimensions, including duration, timing, and quality. Moreover, differences in biology, environment, and culture create dramatic intraindividual and interindividual variability. Sleep promotes health through multiple pathways. Sleep enhances learning and cognition and regulates hormonal rhythms and behaviors.[2–5] Sleep also strengthens the immune system.[6,7] Sleep plays a crucial role in early brain development in infants and children. By 2 years of age, children will have spent more time asleep than awake (approximately 14 months asleep vs 10 months awake).

The development of sleep in children is best understood as an interaction between cultural, physiologic, and environmental factors.[8] Sleep in newborns rapidly evolves in conjunction with the caregiving environment, which provides appropriate feeding and interaction schedules. Conversely, children's sleep habits and temperaments affect their caregivers' sleep environment and schedules.[9] Understanding this complex interaction is essential to determine what is developmentally appropriate regarding the duration, structure, and regulation of sleep in children.

[a] Division of Pediatrics, Cooperman Barnabas Medical Center and Children's Hospital of New Jersey at Newark Beth Israel, New Jersey Medical School, 375 Mount Pleasant Avenue, Suite 105, West Orange, NJ 07052, USA; [b] Division of Pediatrics, Children's Hospital of New Jersey at Newark Beth Israel Hospital, 201 Lyons Avenue, Newark, NJ 07112, USA; [c] Division of Respiratory Diseases, Children's Hospital, Boston, Harvard Medical School, Mailstop 208, 300 Longwood Avenue, Boston, MA 02115, USA
* Corresponding author.
E-mail address: eliot.katz@childrens.harvard.edu

Sleep Med Clin 18 (2023) 123–134
https://doi.org/10.1016/j.jsmc.2023.01.007
1556-407X/23/© 2023 Elsevier Inc. All rights reserved.

MEASURING SLEEP

How and what aspects of sleep are measured is vital, particularly when comparing health outcomes. Subjective methods include structured interviews, parental/self-reports, and questionnaires. Commonly used subjective measures include sleep diaries or logs for extended periods and validated questionnaires, such as the Children's Sleep Habits Questionnaire,[10] the Brief Infant Sleep Questionnaire,[11] the Pediatric Sleep Questionnaire,[11] and the Children's Chronotype Questionnaire.[12] Subjective methods are cost-effective but limited because of issues with compliance and recall biases that may lead to overestimating or underestimating sleep durations or characteristics. For example, parents of older children typically do not know when their child is quietly awake in bed.[13–16]

Commonly used objective methods include direct observation, actigraphy, and polysomnography (PSG). Actigraphy monitors body movements by use of a small device placed on the wrist (or ankle) that uses an accelerometer (measuring movement) and software-based algorithms to differentiate sleep-wake states.[17] Data can be collected over extended periods of time in a natural environment and allow visualization of sleep-wake patterns. However, because actigraphy relies on movement, data collected in this way can be misleading. For example, children sleeping in swings, car seats, or strollers can be misclassified as awake. Conversely, a child who is very still while awake can be misclassified as asleep.[14,18–23] In sleep studies comparing parental reports versus actigraphy, data were comparable for sleep schedule but differed significantly for sleep efficiency.[20,21,24] Comparing PSG and actigraphy showed an 85% to 95% agreement for sleep-wake scoring.[25] PSG measures the constituents of sleep (sleep states) and associated breathing patterns.[26] Scoring sleep stages requires at least 3 channels of EEG for brain activity, electro-oculogram for eye movements, and electromyogram for muscle tone.[27,28] Other parameters calculated include (1) total recording time (the time between lights off and lights on), (2) total sleep time (the total amount of sleep time scored during the total recording time), (3) sleep efficiency (percent of time in bed sleeping), (4) sleep latency (the time it takes to fall asleep after turning the lights out), (5) rapid eye movement (REM) latency (time from sleep onset to the first appearance of an REM episode), and (6) wake after sleep onset.[26] For children, PSG typically consists of 10 to 12 hours of sleep in a quiet, dark room (in a laboratory) with 1 parent at the bedside. Child cooperation is vital, but infants and children may have difficulty falling asleep in a new environment. Given that testing is also expensive, most studies are performed for 1 night, which provides limited data about an individual's day-to-day sleep variability.

Because parent/self-report, direct observations, actigraphy, and PSG have strengths and weaknesses, a combination of these measures is used clinically and in research.

POLYSOMNOGRAPHY NIGHT-TO-NIGHT VARIABILITY

An adaptation effect of the sleep laboratory environment, termed the "first night effect," has been reported to disrupt sleep architecture[29] and perhaps underestimate respiratory disturbances. In 30 children studied between 1 and 4 weeks apart, Katz and colleagues[30] found no significant night-to-night difference in the sleep efficiency, arousal index, or the percentage of REM sleep or nonrapid eye movement (NREM) sleep. Most studies in children have demonstrated excellent consistency in the diagnosis of respiratory abnormalities from night to night.[29–32] The intrasubject respiratory parameters, however, demonstrated considerable variability, particularly in children with severe disease. The variability in respiratory parameters could not be accounted for by changes in body position or percent REM time. However, 2 consecutive nights of home-based sleep testing found that 40% of children with a normal apnea-hypopnea index on night 1 had obstructive sleep apnea on night 2.[33] Thus, clinically important night-to-night variability may be present in some children independent of a "first-night effect." Rebuffat and colleagues[34] demonstrated little night-to-night variability in sleep state or apneas in overnight polysomnograms on 2 to 3 successive nights on 19 term infants.

SLEEP DURATION

Total sleep time is an indicator of sleep need, which has large individual differences. For example, infants have considerable day-to-day variability, in some cases up to 12 hours, in their amount of daily sleep time.[35] Moreover, at 6 months of age, total sleep time ranges from 10.4 to 18 hours.[36] The large variability in awakenings and cultural differences also contributes to individual differences.[21,37–39] For this reason, it is difficult to obtain consensus on the recommended total sleep time for infants from birth to 3 months of age.[40]

On average, term infants sleep about 12 to 17 hours in a 24-hour period.[41] The 2016 consensus statement of the American Academy of Sleep Medicine indicated that less than 12 hours of sleep or more than 18 hours were inappropriate in newborns.[42] Because of an immature circadian rhythm and a robust homeostatic drive, infants have a highly polyphasic sleep pattern that manifests as multiple brief periods of sleep.[43] At 2 weeks of age, the longest sleep period is about 3 to 4 hours followed by 1 to 2 hours of waking.[36,44] This is driven in part by feeding schedules, with infants requiring a meal every 2 to 4 hours (more frequently for breastfed infants).[45–47] As the brain and circadian rhythm mature, wake periods gradually lengthen, and sleep preferentially skews toward the evening.[28,37]

Total sleep duration for infants 4 to 12 months old ranges from 12 to 16 hours.[40,41] Wake periods increase slowly, whereas daytime naps decrease, ranging 2 to 4 naps per day for 20 to 120 minutes.[48] Sleep consolidation at night increases and, by 5 months of age, the sleep period can be as long as 7 hours. Between 6 and 9 months of age, infants start sleeping through the night for 10 to 12 hours.[49] At 12 months of age, daytime sleep has decreased to 28% to 30% compared with 50% at 1 month.[34,47,50,51]

Recommended total sleep time in toddlers (1–3 years old) is 11 to 14 hours.[40,41] In this age group, sleep changes from polyphasic to biphasic. The frequency of daytime naps continues to decrease, with most toddlers taking only a single nap by 18 months of age.[52] Nighttime awakenings are common at this age. Around 10% of toddlers will continue to have 1 nighttime awakening, and half will have nighttime waking once a week.[42] Mothers of typically developing toddlers frequently report sleep problems (20%–40%) at this age.[53] This may be due in part to the toddler becoming more independent around sleep, transitioning from a crib to a bed, and developing nighttime fears.

Recommended total sleep time in preschool children (3–5 years old) is 10 to 13 hours.[40,41] Sleep changes from biphasic to monophasic. Daytime naps vary because they are influenced by individual differences, daycare schedules, parental expectations, family routines, and cultural norms.[54] In 1 study, 50% of toddler's naps lasted for 76 minutes.[54] In general, 81% of 3-year-olds and 41% of 4-year-olds still napped.[18] By age 6, fewer than 10% still napped.[18]

Recommended total sleep time in school-aged children (6–12 years old) is 9 to 12 hours.[40,41] Sleep is consolidated to nighttime and associated with high levels of alertness during the day.[55] School-aged children tend to go to bed and rise early.

Recommended total sleep time in adolescents (12–18 years old) is 8 to 10 hours.[40,41] The decrease in total sleep duration from school age to adolescence is multifactorial, owing in part to changes in circadian rhythms and school start times, as sleep needs are similar.[56]

In summary, total sleep time decreases with decreased daytime sleep, changes from polyphasic to monophasic with the need for daytime naps disappearing for most children by the age of 5 years, and sleep needs remain stable starting at 10 years of age (**Table 1**).

SLEEP ARCHITECTURE AND CYCLING

With age, the quality and quantity of sleep change greatly together, shown by percentage of sleep states and EEG activity patterns. Maturation of electrical activity with brain development follows

Table 1
Developmental changes in sleep duration and patterns: newborns to adolescents

Age	Total sleep time (TST) (h)	Sleep Pattern	Sleep Preference	Length of Sleep Episodes (h)	No. of Naps
Newborns 0–2 mo	14–17	Highly polyphasic	Diurnal = Nocturnal	3–4	—
Infant 3–11 mo	12–16	Polyphasic	Nocturnal > Diurnal	7–9	2–4
Toddler 12–36 mo	11–14	Biphasic	Nocturnal >> Diurnal	7–9	1–2
Preschool 3–5 y-old	10–13	Biphasic	Nocturnal >>> Diurnal	7–9	1
School age 6–12 y-old	6–12	Monophasic	Nocturnal	—	0
Teenager 13–18 y-old	8–10	Monophasic	Nocturnal	—	0

an organized progression, with sleep spindles, K-complexes, and slow-wave activity emerging. Brain development and sleep phenomenology mature at a similar rate, independent of whether the infant is in utero or postdelivery.[43]

In adults, sleep architecture is a highly structured process involving cycling of NREM and REM sleep stages through the night. Interspersed throughout the sleep cycle are brief arousals and awakenings. The final mature pattern, which is present beyond infancy into adolescence, begins in NREM sleep and progresses into REM sleep. Each 90-minute NREM-REM cycle consists of about 80 minutes of NREM sleep followed by 10 minutes of REM sleep. The cycle is repeated about 3 to 6 times during the night (**Fig. 1**).[57] In contrast, sleep in infants often begins in REM and progresses into NREM. Each REM-NREM cycle (45–60 minutes) consists of about 30 minutes of REM sleep followed by 30 minutes of NREM sleep, and the cycle is repeated once or twice before an awakening.[58]

Mature NREM sleep is conventionally divided into 3 stages based on characteristic EEG findings (**Fig. 2**). Overall, NREM sleep is associated with persistent muscle tone and an active regulating brain with increasing arousal thresholds as NREM sleep progresses from stage 1 to 3. Characteristic physiologic changes during NREM sleep include reduced activity; autonomic slowing; maintenance of thermoregulation; episodic, involuntary movements; few REMs; and reduced blood flow.[59]

REM sleep is not divided into stages; rather, there are 2 phases: tonic and phasic. Overall, REM sleep is characterized by wakelike, high-frequency, low-amplitude, and decreased synchronized EEG

activity; episodic bursts of saccades of quick conjugate eye movements; and absent chin tone representing muscle atonia with intermittent muscle twitching. Characteristic physiologic changes during REM sleep include autonomic activation, altered thermoregulation, and skeletal muscle paralysis.[59]

DEVELOPMENT OF SLEEP STATES

The behavioral correlates of wakefulness, active sleep or REM sleep, and quiet sleep or NREM sleep appear around 28 to 30 weeks' conceptional age, but not by EEG criteria. The EEG is still undifferentiated reflecting the immature nervous system. A recognizable EEG pattern of REM and NREM sleep first appears at 30 to 32 weeks.[60] Transitional or indeterminate sleep is also evident, characterized by discordant features of EEG, electro-oculogram, chin electromyogram, respiration, and body movements.[61] By 37 to 38 weeks, the EEG activity in wakefulness and REM sleep is similar in appearance. Moreover, because sleep often begins with REM sleep, it is difficult to determine when an infant has transitioned from wake to sleep; thus, behavioral correlates (such as eye closure for longer than 3 minutes) are used to differentiate between these 2 states.[28] By 3 to 4 months of age, waking EEG becomes more distinct via the dominant posterior rhythm (DPR), and the frequency then increases from around 4 Hz at 4 months to 8 Hz by 3 years of age. The DPR is present in the wakeful state when the eyes are closed and attenuates with eye opening.[62]

By 3 months of age, the 3 stages of NREM sleep can be distinguished. Stage 2 NREM is defined by 1- to 3-second bursts of asynchronous spindle

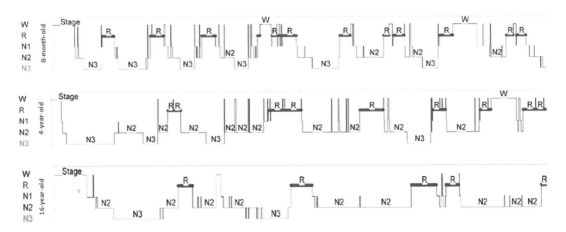

Fig. 1. Hypnogram from an 8-month-old, 4-year-old, and 16-year-old demonstrating changes in slow-wave sleep (N3 NREM) and REM sleep, which is maximal in infants and decreases with age. N1, stage 1 NREM sleep; N2, stage 2 NREM sleep; N3, stage 3 NREM sleep; R, REM; W, wake.

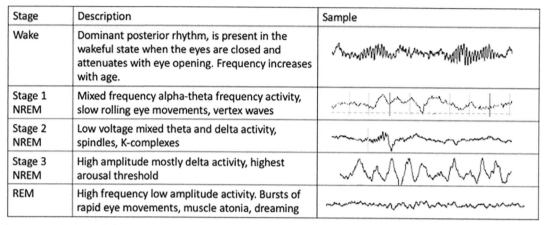

Stage	Description	Sample
Wake	Dominant posterior rhythm, is present in the wakeful state when the eyes are closed and attenuates with eye opening. Frequency increases with age.	
Stage 1 NREM	Mixed frequency alpha-theta frequency activity, slow rolling eye movements, vertex waves	
Stage 2 NREM	Low voltage mixed theta and delta activity, spindles, K-complexes	
Stage 3 NREM	High amplitude mostly delta activity, highest arousal threshold	
REM	High frequency low amplitude activity. Bursts of rapid eye movements, muscle atonia, dreaming	

Fig. 2. Description of sleep stages.

activity (12–15 Hz), which appears at 2 to 3 months of age; 50% of sleep spindles are synchronous by 6 and 9 months of age, and 70% are synchronous by 12 months of age.[63] Delayed appearance or abnormal-appearing sleep spindles are an early biomarker of a metabolic and/or brain abnormality.[63] K-complexes and vertex waves typically appear at about 5 months of age and are well established by 18 months. Stage 3 NREM usually appears between 3 and 6 months. Sleep begins with REM sleep until about 3 to 6 months of age, when it then begins with NREM. [29,62]At 6 months of age, stage 3 NREM sleep is preferentially present toward the beginning of the night and REM sleep is preferentially present in the latter half.[48,64]

After 1 year of age, sleep architecture continues to become more defined. NREM sleep occupies about 51% to 61% of total sleep time, and REM sleep occupies about 26% to 40%.[48] REM onset latency increases, and REM starts to show atonia (absence of muscle movements).[27] Sleep efficiency increases around 12 to 24 months of age, in part because of a higher arousal threshold.[27] By age 12 years, sleep architecture resembles that of adults. **Table 2** summarizes the development of specific EEG features of sleep and wake.

An important change during the first few years of life is the marked decrease in REM sleep.[65] From term until 3 months of age, REM sleep comprises 50% to 60% of total sleep time. After 3 months of age, REM sleep comprises 34% to 50% of total sleep time. By 1 year, REM sleep comprises only 20% to 30% of total sleep time.[65] The functional significance of this change is unclear, but the time course of REM sleep development and decline corresponds to important periods of brain maturation.[63,66]

Several normal EEG patterns can be seen during sleep in children and not in adults. Although discussion of these EEG patterns is beyond the

scope of this article, they include anterior slow-wave activity, hypnagogic hypersynchrony, hypersynchronous theta, postarousal hypersynchrony, rhythmic anterior theta activity of drowsiness, and the frontal arousal rhythm.[62]

In summary, rapid and progressive changes in sleep phenomenology are seen in the first decade of life, with the development of distinct behavioral states: REM, NREM, and wakefulness. These states are characterized by a recurring and relatively stable pattern of physiologic and behavioral changes that represent distinct modes of central nervous system maturation and reorganization.

SLEEP REGULATION

In 1982, Borbely[67] developed a practical theoretic model suggesting that sleep is regulated by a sleep-wake–dependent homeostatic process (process S) and a clocklike circadian process (process C). Process S is a "sleep pressure" that builds during waking hours and is relieved by sleep. In addition to contributing to "sleep pressure," process C dictates the timing, duration, and structure of sleep.[68] These 2 processes are distinct and function independently from 1 another, but together allow for the consolidation of a sustained bout of wakefulness during the daytime hours and a nocturnal sleep episode of good depth and duration.

The homeostatic system currently has no clear single "center," like the suprachiasmatic nucleus is for the circadian system. During the day, homeostatic drive (sleep pressure) builds with every hour of sustained wakefulness until a critical point is reached. This then allows for rapid sleep initiation and deep, slow-wave sleep. In sleep, with each passing NREM-REM cycle, the sleep homeostatic drive is partially dispelled. Sleep latency and slow-wave activity (power density in the 0.75- to

Table 2
Developmental changes of sleep/wake electroencephalogram from infants to adolescence

Age	Sleep Onset	NREM-REM Cycle Length	Dominant Posterior Rhythm	Sleep Spindles	Vertex Waves and K-Complexes
Newborns 0-2 mo	REM sleep onset	50–60 min	Not present	12–14 Hz first seen at 44–46 post-conceptional age (CA)	Not present
Infant 3–11 mo	NREM sleep	—	5–6 Hz	Asynchronous to 70% synchronized by 11 mo	K-complex appears at 5–6 mo
Toddler 12–36 mo	NREM sleep	—	6–8 Hz	12–15 Hz	Mature vertex waves by 16 mo
Preschool 3–5 y-old	NREM sleep	85–115 min	8 Hz	12–15 Hz	K-complexes occur in rapid runs
School age 6–12 y-old	NREM sleep	—	10 Hz	12–15 Hz, sleep spindles often associated with K-complexes	K-complexes maximal frontal, vertex waves central
Teenager 13–18 y-old	NREM sleep	90 min	10 Hz	Frontal spindles until 13 y-old	K-complexes maximal frontal, vertex waves central

4.5-Hz frequency) are markers of the strength of the sleep homeostatic drive.[69] Process C promotes arousal during the daytime and sleep during the night. Central to the circadian process is the master circadian oscillator found in the suprachiasmatic nucleus of the hypothalamus.[70] Primary environmental cues (zeitgebers) entrain and synchronize internal processes, such as the sleep-wake patterns, core body temperature, and pineal melatonin production to the 24-hour day. Environmental light is the major zeitgeber. Light is transmitted through a class of retinal ganglion cells and to the suprachiasmatic nucleus via the retino-hypothalamic tract. The output of the suprachiasmatic nucleus to the pineal gland promotes the release of melatonin. Melatonin levels increase before sleep, peak during the early morning hours, and drop to low daytime levels just after morning awakening. This pattern of melatonin secretion is used to quantify the timing of the circadian clock.[71] Circadian melatonin phase (ie, dim light melatonin onset; DLMO) is a well-established phase marker of the circadian rhythm. Blood or salivary specimens are obtained frequently throughout a 24-hour period, and the DLMO is defined as the time when melatonin levels increase above a specific threshold. DLMO corresponds to the onset of sleep time. The phase angle of entrainment is defined as the time between the circadian phase and the time of bedtime, midpoint sleep, or rise time.[70–72]

The developmental course of the homeostatic process in infants is not well studied. This is due to the following: (1) inability to "decouple" the

circadian process from the homeostatic process using forced desynchrony paradigms as is done in adolescents[73]; (2) sleep rebound, a marker of the homeostatic process, is measured by slow (delta) wave activity and can only be measured at an age when delta activity is expressed, which occurs around 2 months of age[74]; and (3) longitudinal studies with 24-hour EEG are difficult to perform on healthy newborn infants. In rat models, compensated sleep deprivation with increased time spent in quiet sleep (QS) occurred only later in development.[58] Moreover, the decline in slow-wave activity was seen within a single sleep episode, indicating a shorter time scale for dissipation of sleep pressure.[74,75] Jenni and colleagues[74] speculate that in infants less than 2 months of age, theta activity may be a useful marker of the homeostatic process. Furthermore, the rapid increase and dissipation of sleep pressure and misalignment of the homeostatic system with the circadian system cause the polyphasic sleep patterns seen in newborns. With age, the alignment of the homeostatic system with the circadian system results in sleep consolidation at night.[55] Taken together, research indicates that the homeostatic process may exhibit a different developmental profile in newborns.

Circadian rhythms during the fetal period are linked to maternal entraining signals (rest-activity cycle, heart rate, cortisol, melatonin, and body temperature rhythms). Newborns have no rest-activity circadian rhythm independent of their mother before 1 month of age. Mirmiran and colleagues[76] measured the presence or absence of a circadian rhythm in a group of 40 preterm infants by calculating the magnitude of body temperature range for each infant as they aged. They found the amplitude increased at 3 months of age and remained increased at 6 months of age. However, other research has shown the presence of a circadian rhythm appearing earlier.[77] This discrepancy may be due to the many factors influencing the circadian rhythm, such as feeding (scheduled vs on-demand, breast milk vs formula), environmental lighting (indoor vs outdoor, regular vs irregular light-dark cycle), and chronologic/postconceptional age.[76,78] Less well studied is the role of melatonin found in breast milk, which can influence the development of the circadian rhythm. For example, the change from breast milk to formula or milk pumped during the day (which lacks maternal melatonin) and given at nighttime will attenuate the melatonin peak in maternal milk, which is usually between midnight and 4 AM[79] Infants develop their melatonin rhythm at about 3 months of age, reinforcing the finding that circadian rhythms are usually absent before then.[76]

Homeostatic and circadian processes are thought to continue to develop between 1 and 10 years of age, yet there is little research in this area. Indirect evidence for maturation of the homeostatic process includes the following: (1) a decrease in sleep duration due in part to reduced daytime sleep; (2) decreases in duration and frequency of naps associated with increased nap sleep-onset latencies; and (3) naps dropping out (when they do) at later and later times in the day.[18,36,54,55] Jenni and LeBourgeois[55] argue that younger children accumulate sleep pressure more rapidly than older children and, thus, require naps. The age when children drop their nap is multifactorial and depends on biological and environmental variables (eg, parental and daycare/school schedules). Lassonde and colleagues[80] found that in toddlers who miss their daytime nap, onset of nighttime sleep latency is decreased, and nighttime sleep duration is increased compared with a night following a daytime nap.

Chronotype is a construction reflecting individual differences in diurnal preference (evening vs morning) and is assessed with questionnaires.[81] In toddlers, although there is substantial interindividual difference, there is a relative preference for morning. Moreover, chronotype is linked to the timing of DLMO.[82] LeBourgeois and colleagues[83] studied healthy children 30 to 36 months old with no reported sleep problems and found substantial individual difference with an average DLMO of 7:40 PM ± 48 minutes, which occurred 29 minutes ± 32 minutes before bedtime. They

also found that DLMO was moderately correlated with bedtime and sleep onset time. For example, children with later DLMOs were likely to take longer to fall asleep after lights out, and children who were put to bed closer to their DLMO had longer sleep-onset latencies and increased bedtime resistance.[84] These findings support evidence for the "forbidden zone" of sleep—when sleep is attempted at too early of a circadian time. Thus, they concluded that inappropriate bedtimes relative to a child's circadian phase may contribute to settling difficulties in toddlers.[84]

In adolescents, accumulation of sleep pressure slows, and so staying awake longer is easier.[56,85,86] With regard to the homeostatic process, the recovery sleep process does not change across adolescence; thus, the need for sleep remains stable. Changes in the circadian system mirror the changes in the homeostatic process. Roenneberg and colleagues[87] measured the phase preference or behavioral phase changes with age by measuring the time of the weekend mid sleep, or the middle of the sleep episode when there is nothing constraining sleep. During the ages of 10 to 20 years, this middle of sleep gets later and later. This shift may be explained by the following facts. First, there is a progressive delay or later timing amount of the melatonin onset phase. This phase delay may be due to change in light exposure in adolescents, who tend to stay up later and wake up later. Second, the intrinsic circadian period is longer than that in adults. Last, the amplitude of the circadian rhythm diminishes.[56,85,88–91] Overall, sleep regulation processes in adolescents, along with environmental pressures, such as nightly homework and sport activities, encourage later bedtimes, but early school start times often lead to sleep restriction.

SLEEP RESPIRATORY ONTOGENY

At birth, the high compliance of the infant's chest wall results in very low end-expiratory volume, and therefore, low oxygen reserve. The lung volumes in infants decrease approximately 30% further during REM sleep, rendering them particularly vulnerable to oxygen desaturation.[92] Consequently, oxygen desaturations are commonly observed in infants with even brief respiratory pauses during REM sleep. By contrast, older infants (beyond 0.5–1 year) have lower chest wall compliance, a higher end-expiratory volume, and therefore, sufficient oxygen reserve to sustain oxygen saturations during normal respiratory pauses.

The baseline oxygen saturation during sleep in a healthy term infant has a median of 97.9%, with the 10th percentile of 95.2%.[93] However, 59% of infants had at least one 3-minute epoch with a baseline oxygen saturation less than 90%.[93] Furthermore, the median oxygen saturation nadir in a healthy term infant is 83%, with the 10th percentile being 78%.[93] By contrast, oxygen desaturation is only occasionally observed during respiratory pauses in older children.[94] Moss and colleagues[95] reported that only 18% of children (aged 10.1 ± 0.7) experienced an oxygen desaturation below 90%. Overall, central apneas defined as ≥20 seconds or associated with a 4% oxygen desaturation are generally recorded less than 1 per hour in normal children.[96,97]

The mean airway closing pressure for infants at 2 months of age is −0.5 cm H_2O under anesthesia and is −0.7 ± 2 cm H_2O in postmortem studies.[98] The infant upper airway is so highly compliant that a 2 cm H_2O change in luminal pressure results in a 50% reduction in cross-sectional area.[99] Thus, the infant airway closing pressure is very close to atmospheric pressure, indicating a high risk for collapse during sleep. During the first year of life, the infant's airway becomes more stable with a reduction in the passive closing pressure to −6 cm H_2O.[99] During NREM sleep, however, the closing pressure in infants is << −25 cm H_2O,[100] indicating the effectiveness of neuromuscular activation to sustain pharyngeal patency in this sleep state.

Obstructive apnea or mixed apnea appears to be more common in premature infants and decreases in frequency over the first year of life. In thermistor-based studies, Guilleminault and colleagues[101] reported that obstructive apneas in term infants occur 0.62 per hour at 3 weeks, 1.14 per hour at 6 weeks, 0.43 per hour at 3 months, and 0.20 per hour at 6 months; Hoppenbrouwers and colleagues[102] reported that obstructive apneas in term infants occurred 0.68 per hour at 1 month, 0.57 per hour at 3 months, and 0.22 per hour at 6 months. Using nasal pressure recordings, Daftary and colleagues[103] studied 30 term infants at approximately 20 days of age and reported a mean obstructive apnea index of 2.3 per /hour and the mean oxygen saturation nadir of 84% ± 4.8%.

In older children (mean, 9.7 ± 4.6 years), Marcus and colleagues[104] presented the respiratory data during sleep in 50 children, and 9 had at least 1 obstructive apneic event. Only 15% of normal children had any hypopneas with the mean hypopnea index being 0.1 ± 0.1 (range, 0.1–0.7).[105] Acebo and colleagues[106] also reported that hypopneas were rare in older children and adolescents. Montgomery-Downs and colleagues[107] studied 542 healthy children between 3.2 and 8.6 years of age and found an average obstructive apnea index of 0.03 per hour in the younger half and 0.05 per hour in their older children. Thus, in older children, an obstructive apnea-hypopnea index greater than 1 per hour is considered to be statistically abnormal, although the clinical significance of this threshold level has not been established.

SUMMARY

During the first 2 decades, multiple important changes in sleep patterns and organization mirror brain maturation and development. The transitions are dramatic. Infants spend more time asleep than awake. By around 9 months of age, total sleep time decreases, with nocturnal sleep consolidation developing. By 5 years of age, daytime sleep time decreases with the need for naps ceasing. Sleep phenomenology flips with more than half in REM stage sleep in newborns changing to more than half of NREM stage sleep in adolescents. Sleep cycle length increases from 60 minutes in infancy to 90 to 120 minutes in adolescents. Sleep regulation develops with sleep phase preference to the morning during school age and sleep phase delays in adolescence. Last, individual variations in all these domains are enormous because of the bidirectional interactions of genetic, environmental, and cultural influences.

Respiratory parameters change when asleep and are state dependent. Infants have a more collapsible upper airway and lower lung volumes than older children, which predisposes them to obstructive sleep apnea and sleep-related hypoxemia. Infants also have ventilatory control instability with a narrow difference between the baseline eupneic carbon dioxide level and the apneic threshold, resulting in periodic breathing until approximately 6 months of age. Maturation of chest wall mechanics is mostly complete by 6 months of age, and airway collapsibility decreases to levels seen in older children by 1 year of age.

CLINICS CARE POINTS

- Many children present with reported difficulty initiating or maintaining sleep, but are able to awaken easily in the morning and are otherwise asymptomatic. Consider the possibility that these children are constitutionally short sleepers who are simply being put to bed too early.

- Although many adolescents report sleeping only 7 to 8 hours per night, only a subset of these children will present with sleepiness. Consider the possibility that these sleepy adolescents are getting chronically insufficient sleep and need therapeutic extension in their sleep duration.

- Hypoxemia is commonly observed in infants related to periodic breathing and increased chest wall compliance resulting in low lung volumes. These predispositions typically resolve by 6 months, as does the hypoxemia.

CONFLICTS OF INTEREST

No conflicts of interests with any of the authors.

REFERENCES

1. Siegel J. Principles and practice of sleep medicine. In: Kryger MH, Roth T, Goldstein CA, et al, editors. [Kryger, 2022 #181]. Seventh edition. Philadelphia, PA: Elsevier; 2022. p. 52–3.
2. Beebe DW. Cognitive, behavioral, and functional consequences of inadequate sleep in children and adolescents. Pediatr Clin North Am 2011; 58(3):649–65.
3. Dahl RE. The impact of inadequate sleep on children's daytime cognitive function. Semin Pediatr Neurol 1996;3(1):44–50.
4. Vriend J, Davidson F, Rusak B, et al. Emotional and cognitive impact of sleep restriction in children. Sleep Med Clin 2015;10(2):107–15.
5. Vriend JL, Davidson FD, Corkum PV, et al. Manipulating sleep duration alters emotional functioning and cognitive performance in children. J Pediatr Psychol 2013;38(10):1058–69.
6. Irwin MR, Opp MR. Sleep health: reciprocal regulation of sleep and innate immunity. Neuropsychopharmacology 2017;42(1):129–55.
7. Poluektov MG. Sleep and immunity. Neurosci Behav Physiol 2021;1–7.
8. Jenni OG, O'Connor BB. Children's sleep: an interplay between culture and biology. Pediatrics 2005; 115(1 Suppl):204–16.
9. Sadeh A, Mindell JA. Infant sleep interventions - Methodological and conceptual issues. Sleep Med Rev 2016;29:123–5. https://doi.org/10.1016/j.smrv.2015.11.002.
10. Owens JA, Spirito A, McGuinn M. The Children's Sleep Habits Questionnaire (CSHQ): psychometric properties of a survey instrument for school-aged children. Sleep 2000;23(8):1043–51. Available at: http://www.ncbi.nlm.nih.gov/pubmed/11145319.
11. Sadeh A. A brief screening questionnaire for infant sleep problems: validation and findings for an Internet sample. Pediatrics 2004;113(6):e570–7.
12. Chervin RD, Hedger K, Dillon JE, Pituch KJ. Pediatric sleep questionnaire (PSQ): validity and reliability of scales for sleep-disordered breathing, snoring, sleepiness, and behavioral problems. Sleep Med 2000;1(1):21–32.
13. Arnardottir ES, Islind AS, Oskarsdottir M. The Future of Sleep Measurements: A Review and Perspective. Sleep Med Clin 2021;16(3):447–64.
14. Sen T, Spruyt K. Pediatric Sleep Tools: An Updated Literature Review. Front Psychiatry 2020;11:317.
15. Spruyt K, Gozal D. Pediatric sleep questionnaires as diagnostic or epidemiological tools: a review of currently available instruments. Sleep Med Rev 2011;15(1):19–32.
16. Stražišar BG. Sleep Measurement in Children-Are We on the Right Track? Sleep Med Clin 2021; 16(4):649–60 (In eng).
17. Ancoli-Israel S, Martin JL, Blackwell T, et al. The SBSM Guide to Actigraphy Monitoring: Clinical and Research Applications. Behav Sleep Med 2015;13(Suppl 1):S4–38.
18. Acebo C, Sadeh A, Seifer R, Tzischinsky O, Hafer A, Carskadon MA. Sleep/wake patterns derived from activity monitoring and maternal report for healthy 1- to 5-year-old children. Sleep 2005;28(12):1568–77 (In eng).
19. Acebo C, Sadeh A, Seifer R, et al. Estimating sleep patterns with activity monitoring in children and adolescents: how many nights are necessary for reliable measures? Sleep 1999;22(1):95–103 (In eng).
20. Camerota M, Tully KP, Grimes M, Gueron-Sela N, Propper CB. Assessment of infant sleep: how well do multiple methods compare? Sleep 2018; 41(10). https://doi.org/10.1093/sleep/zsy146.
21. Hall WA, Liva S, Moynihan M, Saunders R. A comparison of actigraphy and sleep diaries for infants' sleep behavior. Front Psychiatry 2015;6:19.
22. Sadeh A, Acebo C. The role of actigraphy in sleep medicine. Sleep Med Rev 2002;6(2):113–24.
23. Sadeh A, Dark I, Vohr BR. Newborns' sleep-wake patterns: the role of maternal, delivery and infant factors. Early Hum Dev 1996;44(2):113–26.
24. Sadeh A. Evaluating night wakings in sleep-disturbed infants: a methodological study of parental reports and actigraphy. Sleep 1996; 19(10):757–62.
25. Sadeh A. Commentary: comparing actigraphy and parental report as measures of children's sleep. J Pediatr Psychol 2008;33(4):406–7.
26. Berry RB, Quan SF, Abreu AR, et al. The AASM Manual for the Scoring of Sleep and Associated Events: Rules, Terminology and Technical Specifications. Darien, IL: American Academy of Sleep Medicine; 2020.
27. Grigg-Damberger M, Gozal D, Marcus CL, et al. The visual scoring of sleep and arousal in infants and children. J Clin Sleep Med 2007;3(2):201–40. Available at: https://www.ncbi.nlm.nih.gov/pubmed/17557427.

28. Grigg-Damberger MM. The Visual Scoring of Sleep in Infants 0 to 2 Months of Age. J Clin Sleep Med 2016;12(3):429–45.

29. Scholle S, Scholle HC, Kemper A, et al. First night effect in children and adolescents undergoing polysomnography for sleep-disordered breathing. Clinical neurophysiology 2003;114(11):2138–45.

30. Katz ES, Greene MG, Carson KA, et al. Night-to-night variability of polysomnography in children with suspected obstructive sleep apnea. The Journal of pediatrics 2002;140(5):589–94.

31. Li AM, Wing YK, Cheung A, et al. Is a 2-Night Polysomnographic Study Necessary in Childhood Sleep-Related Disordered Breathing? Chest 2004; 126(5):1467–72.

32. Verhulst SL, Schrauwen N, De Backer WA, Desager KN. First night effect for polysomnographic data in children and adolescents with suspected sleep disordered breathing. Archives of disease in childhood 2006;91(3):233–7.

33. Ørntoft M, Andersen IG, Homøe P. Night-to-night variability in respiratory parameters in children and adolescents examined for obstructive sleep apnea. International journal of pediatric otorhinolaryngology 2020;137:110206.

34. Rebuffat E, Groswasser J, Kelmanson I, et al. Polygraphic evaluation of night-to-night variability in sleep characteristics and apneas in infants. Sleep 1994;17(4):329–32.

35. Wooding AR, Boyd J, Geddis DC. Sleep patterns of New Zealand infants during the first 12 months of life. J Paediatr Child Health 1990;26(2):85–8.

36. Galland BC, Taylor BJ, Elder DE, Herbison P. Normal sleep patterns in infants and children: a systematic review of observational studies. Sleep Med Rev 2012;16(3):213–22.

37. Anders TF, Keener M. Developmental course of nighttime sleep-wake patterns in full-term and premature infants during the first year of life. I. Sleep 1985;8(3):173–92.

38. Caudill W, Plath DW. Who Sleeps by Whom? Parent-Child Involvement in Urban Japanese Families (dagger). Psychiatry 1966;29(4):344–66.

39. Morelli GA, Rogoff B, Oppenheim D, Goldsmith D. Cultural Variation in Infants' Sleeping Arrangements. Developmental Psychology 1992;28(4): 604–13.

40. Paruthi S, Brooks LJ, D'Ambrosio C, et al. Recommended Amount of Sleep for Pediatric Populations: A Consensus Statement of the American Academy of Sleep Medicine. J Clin Sleep Med 2016;12(6): 785–6.

41. Hirshkowitz M, Whiton K, Albert SM, et al. National Sleep Foundation's sleep time duration recommendations: methodology and results summary. Sleep Health 2015;1(1):40–3.

42. Paruthi S, Brooks LJ, D'Ambrosio C, et al. Consensus Statement of the American Academy of Sleep Medicine on the Recommended Amount of Sleep for Healthy Children: Methodology and Discussion. J Clin Sleep Med 2016;12(11): 1549–61.

43. Lamblin MD, Walls Esquivel E, André M. The electroencephalogram of the full-term newborn: Review of normal features and hypoxic-ischemic encephalopathy patterns. Neurophysiologie clinique 2013; 43(5):267–87.

44. Parmelee AH Jr, Wenner WH, Schulz HR. Infant Sleep Patterns: From Birth to 16 Weeks of Age. J Pediatr 1964;65:576–82.

45. Elias MF, Nicolson NA, Bora C, Johnston J. Sleep/wake patterns of breast-fed infants in the first 2 years of life. Pediatrics 1986;77(3):322–9.

46. Walker AM, Menaham S. Normal early infant behaviour patterns. J Paediatr Child Health 1994; 30(3):260–2.

47. Weinraub M, Bender RH, Friedman SL, et al. Patterns of developmental change in infants' nighttime sleep awakenings from 6 through 36 months of age. Dev Psychol 2012;48(6):1511–28.

48. Burnham MM, Goodlin-Jones BL, Gaylor EE, Anders TF. Nighttime sleep-wake patterns and self-soothing from birth to one year of age: a longitudinal intervention study. J Child Psychol Psychiatry 2002;43(6):713–25.

49. Anders TF, Halpern LF, Hua J. Sleeping through the night: a developmental perspective. Pediatrics 1992;90(4):554–60. Available at: https://www.ncbi.nlm.nih.gov/pubmed/1408509.

50. Sadeh A, Mindell JA, Luedtke K, Wiegand B. Sleep and sleep ecology in the first 3 years: a web-based study. J Sleep Res 2009;18(1):60–73.

51. So K, Adamson TM, Horne RS. The use of actigraphy for assessment of the development of sleep/wake patterns in infants during the first 12 months of life. J Sleep Res 2007;16(2):181–7.

52. Iglowstein I, Jenni OG, Molinari L, Largo RH. Sleep duration from infancy to adolescence: reference values and generational trends. Pediatrics 2003; 111(2):302–7.

53. Owens JA, Witmans M. Sleep problems. Current problems in pediatric and adolescent health care 2004;34(4):154–79.

54. Ward TM, Gay C, Anders TF, Alkon A, Lee KA. Sleep and napping patterns in 3-to-5 year old children attending full-day childcare centers. J Pediatr Psychol 2008;33(6):666–72.

55. Jenni OG, LeBourgeois MK. Understanding sleep-wake behavior and sleep disorders in children: the value of a model. Curr Opin Psychiatry 2006;19(3): 282–7.

56. Carskadon MA. Sleep in adolescents: the perfect storm. Pediatr Clin North Am 2011;58(3):637–47.

57. Edward FP-S, Hobson JA. The Neurobiology of Sleep: Genetics, Cellular Physiology and Subcortical Networks. Nature reviews Neuroscience 2002;3(8):591.
58. Blumberg MS, Gall AJ, Todd WD. The Development of Sleep-Wake Rhythms and the Search for Elemental Circuits in the Infant Brain. Behavioral neuroscience 2014;128(3):250–63.
59. Berry RB, Wagner MH. Introduction. Sleep Medicine Pearls2015:64-68.
60. Curzi-Dascalova L, Peirano P, Morel-Kahn F. Development of sleep states in normal premature and full-term newborns. Developmental psychobiology 1988;21(5):431–44.
61. Dreyfus-Brisac C. Ontogenesis of sleep in human prematures after 32 weeks of conceptional age. Developmental psychobiology 1970;3(2):91–121.
62. Marcuse LV, Fields MC, Yoo J. The normal EEG from neonates to adolescents. Rowan's Primer of EEG; 2016. p. 67–86.
63. Grigg-Damberger MM. Ontogeny of sleep and its functions in infancy, childhood and adolescence. In: Nevšímalová S, Bruni O, editors. Sleep Disorders in Children. Springer International Publishing Switzerland; 2017.
64. Louis J, Cannard C, Bastuji H, Challamel MJ. Sleep ontogenesis revisited: a longitudinal 24-hour home polygraphic study on 15 normal infants during the first two years of life. Sleep 1997;20(5):323–33.
65. Roffwarg HP, Muzio JN, Dement WC. Ontogenetic Development of the Human Sleep-Dream Cycle. Science (American Association for the Advancement of Science) 1966;152(3722):604–19.
66. Sheldon SH. Development of Sleep in Infants and Children. Principles and Practice of Pediatric Sleep Medicine 2014;17–23.
67. Borbely AA. A two process model of sleep regulation. Hum Neurobiol 1982;1(3):195–204. Available at: https://www.ncbi.nlm.nih.gov/pubmed/7185792.
68. Dijk DJ, Czeisler CA. Contribution of the circadian pacemaker and the sleep homeostat to sleep propensity, sleep structure, electroencephalographic slow waves, and sleep spindle activity in humans. Journal of neuroscience 1995;15(5):3526–38.
69. Borbély AA, Achermann P. Sleep homeostasis and models of sleep regulation. Journal of biological rhythms 1999;14(6):557–68.
70. Wyatt JK. Circadian rhythm sleep disorders. Pediatr Clin North Am 2011;58(3):621–35.
71. Markov D, Goldman M. Normal sleep and circadian rhythms: neurobiologic mechanisms underlying sleep and wakefulness. Psychiatr Clin North Am 2006;29(4):841–53. abstract vii.
72. Carskadon MA, Acebo C, Richardson GS, Tate BA, Seifer R. An approach to studying circadian rhythms of adolescent humans. J Biol Rhythms 1997;12(3):278–89.
73. Carskadon MA, Labyak SE, Acebo C, Seifer R. Intrinsic circadian period of adolescent humans measured in conditions of forced desynchrony. Neurosci Lett 1999;260(2):129–32 (In eng).
74. Jenni OG, Borbely AA, Achermann P. Development of the nocturnal sleep electroencephalogram in human infants. American Journal of Physiology - Regulatory, Integrative and Comparative Physiology 2004;286(3):528–38.
75. Frank MG, Morrissette R, Heller HC. Effects of sleep deprivation in neonatal rats. American Journal of Physiology - Regulatory, Integrative and Comparative Physiology 1998;275(1):148–57.
76. Mirmiran M, Maas YG, Ariagno RL. Development of fetal and neonatal sleep and circadian rhythms. Sleep Med Rev 2003;7(4):321–34.
77. McGraw K, Hoffmann R, Harker C, Herman JH. The development of circadian rhythms in a human infant. Sleep (New York, NY) 1999;22(3):303–10.
78. Mirmiran M, Baldwin RB, Ariagno RL. Circadian and sleep development in preterm infants occurs independently from the influences of environmental lighting. Pediatr Res 2003;53(6):933–8.
79. Sadeh A. Sleep and melatonin in infants: A preliminary study. Sleep (New York, NY) 1997;20(3):185–91.
80. Lassonde JM, Rusterholz T, Kurth S, Schumacher AM, Achermann P, LeBourgeois MK. Sleep Physiology in Toddlers: Effects of Missing a Nap on Subsequent Night Sleep. Neurobiol Sleep Circadian Rhythms 2016;1(1):19–26.
81. Werner H, Lebourgeois MK, Geiger A, Jenni OG. Assessment of chronotype in four- to eleven-year-old children: reliability and validity of the Children's Chronotype Questionnaire (CCTQ). Chronobiol Int 2009;26(5):992–1014.
82. Simpkin CT, Jenni OG, Carskadon MA, et al. Chronotype is associated with the timing of the circadian clock and sleep in toddlers. J Sleep Res 2014;23(4):397–405.
83. LeBourgeois MK, Carskadon MA, Akacem LD, et al. Circadian phase and its relationship to nighttime sleep in toddlers. J Biol Rhythms 2013;28(5):322–31.
84. Lebourgeois MK, Wright KP Jr, Lebourgeois HB, Jenni OG. Dissonance Between Parent-Selected Bedtimes and Young Children's Circadian Physiology Influences Nighttime Settling Difficulties. Mind Brain Educ 2013;7(4):234–42.
85. Crowley SJ, Acebo C, Fallone G, Carskadon MA. Estimating dim light melatonin onset (DLMO) phase in adolescents using summer or school-year sleep/wake schedules. Sleep 2006;29(12):1632–41 (In eng).
86. Jenni OG, Achermann P, Carskadon MA. Homeostatic sleep regulation in adolescents. Sleep 2005;28(11):1446–54.

87. Roenneberg T, Kuehnle T, Pramstaller PP, et al. A marker for the end of adolescence. Curr Biol 2004;14(24):R1038–9.

88. Carskadon MA, Acebo C, Jenni OG. Regulation of adolescent sleep: implications for behavior. Ann N Y Acad Sci 2004;1021:276–91.

89. Carskadon MA, Vieira C, Acebo C. Association between puberty and delayed phase preference. Sleep 1993;16(3):258–62.

90. Carskadon MA, Wolfson AR, Acebo C, Tzischinsky O, Seifer R. Adolescent sleep patterns, circadian timing, and sleepiness at a transition to early school days. Sleep 1998;21(8):871–81. Available at: http://www.ncbi.nlm.nih.gov/pubmed/9871949.

91. Crowley SJ, Acebo C, Carskadon MA. Sleep, circadian rhythms, and delayed phase in adolescence. Sleep Med 2007;8(6):602–12.

92. Henderson-Smart DJ, Read DJ. Reduced lung volume during behavioral active sleep in the newborn. J Appl Physiol 1979;46(6):1081–5.

93. Hunt CE, Corwin MJ, Lister G, et al. Longitudinal assessment of hemoglobin oxygen saturation in healthy infants during the first 6 months of age. J Pediatr 1999;135(5):580–6.

94. Poets CF, Stebbens VA, Samuels MP, et al. Oxygen saturation and breathing patterns in children. Pediatrics (Evanston) 1993;92(5):686–90.

95. Moss D, Urschitz MS, Von Bodman A, et al. Reference values for nocturnal home polysomnography in primary schoolchildren. Pediatr Res 2005;58(5):958–65.

96. Uliel S, Tauman R, Greenfeld M, et al. Normal polysomnographic respiratory values in children and adolescents. Chest 2004;125(3):872–8.

97. Verhulst SL, Schrauwen N, Haentjens D, et al. Reference values for sleep-related respiratory variables in asymptomatic European children and adolescents. Pediatr Pulmonol 2007;42(2):159–67.

98. Wilson SL, Thach BT, Brouillette RT, et al. Upper airway patency in the human infant: influence of airway pressure and posture. J Appl Physiol 1980;48(3):500–4.

99. Isono S. Developmental changes of pharyngeal airway patency: implications for pediatric anesthesia. Pediatric anesthesia 2006;16(2):109–22.

100. Marcus CL, Fernandes Do Prado LB, Lutz J, et al. Developmental changes in upper airway dynamics. J Appl Physiol 2004;97(1):98–108.

101. Guilleminault C, Ariagno R, Korobkin R, et al. Mixed and obstructive sleep apnea and near miss for sudden infant death syndrome .2. Comparison of near miss and normal control infants by age. Pediatrics (Evanston) 1979;64(6):882–91.

102. Hoppenbrouwers T, Hodgman JE, Cabal L. Obstructive apnea, associated patterns of movement, heart rate, and oxygenation in infants at low and increased risk for SIDS. Pediatr Pulmonol 1993;15(1):1–12.

103. Daftary AS, Jalou HE, Shively L, et al. Polysomnography reference values in healthy newborns. J Clin Sleep Med 2019;15(3):437–43.

104. Marcus CL, Omlin KJ, Basinki DJ, et al. Normal polysomnographic values for children and adolescents. Am Rev Respir Dis 1992;146(5):1235–9.

105. Witmans MB, Keens TG, Davidson Ward SL, et al. Obstructive hypopneas in children and adolescents: normal values. Am J Respir Crit Care Med 2003;168(12):1540.

106. Acebo C, Millman RP, Rosenberg C, et al. Sleep, breathing, and cephalometrics in older children and young adults. Part I – Normative values. Chest 1996;109(3):664–72 (In eng).

107. Montgomery-Downs HE, O'Brien LM, Gulliver TE, et al. Polysomnographic characteristics in normal preschool and early school-aged children. Pediatrics 2006;117(3):741–53 (In eng).

Insomnia in Infancy, Childhood, and Adolescence

Michal Kahn, PhD[a,b,*]

KEYWORDS

- Insomnia • Sleep • Infants • Children • Adolescents • CBT-I

KEY POINTS

- Insomnia in youth is highly prevalent, disruptive, and persistent.
- Health care providers should consider sleep-wake patterns in all pediatric assessments.
- Cognitive behavior interventions are the first-line treatment of insomnia, with evidence for efficacy and safety in infants, as well as older children and adolescents.
- The use of exogenous melatonin to treat pediatric insomnia is increasing, yet further evidence for long-term safety is warranted.

INTRODUCTION

While adults sleep for approximately 30% of their time, in children this value is estimated at 40%, and infants spend up to 65% of their first year asleep.[1] These vast time investments indicate the imperative role sleep plays in young people's physiologic, cognitive, and emotional development and functioning.[2,3] Yet, despite their high prevalence and maladaptive consequences, sleep-related problems in youth tend to be disregarded and underdiagnosed.[4] A recently published 15-year longitudinal study found that among children with insomnia, the persistence of symptoms into adulthood was the most common developmental trajectory (43%).[5] Knowledge regarding the assessment and management of insomnia is thus imperative for pediatric health care providers aiming to benefit the development and long-term quality of life of youth and their families. This paper reviews the phenomenology, prevalence, assessment, consequences, cause, and treatment of pediatric insomnia. Given the vast evolution of sleep—as well as other domains—during early infancy, through childhood,

and into adolescence, the unique insomnia management aspects of each of these stages in development will be addressed.

PHENOMENOLOGY AND CLASSIFICATION

Insomnia is characterized by persistent difficulties falling asleep, staying asleep, or waking up earlier than desired, resulting in insufficient quality sleep and associated dysfunction and/or distress. Unlike the second edition of the International Classification of Sleep Disorders (ICSD-2),[6] which comprised separate diagnostic entities for adult and childhood insomnia, the third and latest edition incorporates all age groups under the category of "chronic insomnia disorder."[7] The Diagnostic and Statistical Manual of Mental Disorders, Fifth Edition (DSM-5) similarly includes different manifestations of insomnia under a unified diagnostic category, named "insomnia disorder."[8] Criteria in both diagnostic systems dictate that difficulties initiating and maintaining sleep occur at least 3 times per week and that these difficulties and related daytime impairment are experienced for at least 3 months. To qualify for diagnosis, the sleep disturbances

---

[a] School of Psychological Sciences, Tel Aviv University, Tel Aviv, Israel; [b] College of Education, Psychology and Social Work, Flinders University, Sturt Road, Bedford Park, South Australia 5042, Australia
* School of Psychological Sciences, Tel Aviv University, Ramat Aviv 6997801, Israel
E-mail address: michal.kahn@flinders.edu.au

Sleep Med Clin 18 (2023) 135–145
https://doi.org/10.1016/j.jsmc.2023.01.001
1556-407X/23/© 2023 Elsevier Inc. All rights reserved.

should not be better explained by deficient sleep opportunities, inadequate circumstances for sleep (eg, lack of a safe, calm sleep environment), or other coexisting conditions.

In the ICSD-2, pediatric insomnia was described as "behavioral insomnia of childhood" and could be classified into 3 separate subtypes: (1) sleep-onset association type pertained to children whose sleep cues entail external stimuli, such as rocking, patting, breastfeeding, or watching a media screen. This subtype was most common in infants and toddlers and often manifested as multiple nighttime awakenings, given the inability to resume sleep independently following normal nighttime arousal; (2) limit-setting type was more common in older children (toddlers to school-aged) and characterized by bedtime resistance, delays, and tantrums. These were perceived to be a result of parents not setting consistent or sufficient boundaries with regard to their children's sleep; and (3) combined type included both counterproductive sleep associations and bedtime struggles between child and parents.[6] The ICSD-2 additionally included a diagnosis of "psycho-physiological insomnia," which was used to describe difficulties initiating and maintaining sleep as a result of physiologic and mental hyperarousal (eg, racing thoughts), occurring oftentimes in adolescents. Other insomnia subtypes, such as "idiopathic insomnia" and "inadequate sleep hygiene," also appeared in previous editions. However, evidence for poor diagnostic consistency between health care providers[9] led these separate diagnostic entities to be collapsed into a single diagnostic category in the ICSD-3 and DSM-5. Nevertheless, terms such as "sleep-onset association type" are often still used by practitioners to describe the more intricate features of specific insomnia cases.

PREVALENCE

Of the 100+ sleep disorders listed in the ICSD-3, insomnia is by far the most common. Its estimated prevalence in pediatric populations is 10% to 30%.[10] Differences in prevalence estimations found across studies may be a function of the diagnostic criteria used (eg, ICSD-2 vs ICSD-3), assessment methods (eg, clinical interview vs questionnaire), and population characteristics (eg, specific age group). Symptoms are more common in younger compared with older youth, with prevalence approximations as high as 36% in preschool children declining to roughly 11% in adolescents.[11,12] Insomnia is even more ubiquitous in youth diagnosed with neurologic, developmental, or psychiatric disorders.[13] For example, among children diagnosed with autistic spectrum disorder, the prevalence of comorbid insomnia is 60% to 86%, which is 2 to 3 times higher than in typically developing youth.[14] Although there are no differences in prevalence between young boys and girls, a female preponderance emerges from puberty onward.[11] Prevalence rates also vary as a function of regional or cultural factors, with indications of increased parental reporting of insomnia symptoms in predominantly Asian compared with predominantly Caucasian countries.[15]

ASSESSMENT

Pediatric insomnia, as other sleep disorders in youth, tends to be underdiagnosed. Meltzer and colleagues[4] found that only 3.7% of 0 to 18-year-olds attending well-child visits were diagnosed with a sleep disorder—a rate considerably lower than prevalence rates reported in epidemiologic studies. Underdiagnosis may be due to a combination of factors, including limited resources or training, a perception of sleep problems as secondary to other psychiatric conditions (eg, anxiety), or a misconception that youth will surely outgrow these sleep difficulties.[5] Lack of adequate assessment may result in more severe or enduring sleep difficulties, increasing the distress and disfunction of the young person and their family. Hence, it is strongly recommended that any medical or psychiatric evaluation should include an assessment of sleep-wake patterns.

Age-appropriate screening questionnaires, such as the Brief Infant Sleep Questionnaire (BISQ)[16] for infants and toddlers, the Children's Sleep Habits Questionnaire (CSHQ)[17] for preschool and school-aged children, and the Insomnia Severity Index (ISI)[18] for adolescents, can be easily administered in routine health care visits. On indication of sleep difficulties, a clinical interview should be scheduled to characterize the developmental, physiologic, behavioral, and psychosocial aspects and history of the problem. Information should be collected regarding the following: (1) the main complaint, its duration, frequency, history, potential triggers, and previous attempts to address the problem; (2) the youth's typical 24-hour sleep-wake schedule, including sleep-onset latency, sleep onset and offset times, nighttime awakenings, and naps; (3) the consistency of this schedule, particularly between weekdays and weekends. Social jet lag (ie, the sleep debt accumulated during weekdays, which leads to discrepant weekday-weekend sleep timing) may be particularly relevant for adolescents—often indexing a delayed sleep phase disorder; (4) bedtime routines should be described in detail to detect any sleep promoting or hindering activities/agents (eg, bath, media screen exposure); (5) the sleep environment, including room sharing with parents or siblings, noise, temperature, and light conditions; (6) parent-child interactions in the sleep context; (7) medication, caffeine, alcohol, or other substance intake; (8) daytime consequences, including sleepiness and behavior or emotion dysregulation; (9) comorbidities, including other sleep disorders (eg, parasomnias, obstructive sleep apnea, restless legs), mental disorders (eg, anxiety, attention-deficit hyperactivity disorder [ADHD]), or other medical issues (eg, seizures, atopic dermatitis); and finally (10) each family member's current treatment expectations and motivation for change.

In most cases, a thorough clinical interview is sufficient to diagnose insomnia. However, a few additional diagnostic tools may be useful. Sleep diaries—preferably completed for 1 to 2 consecutive weeks—are an accessible way of providing a prospective accurate account of sleep-wake patterns. In recent years, phone applications are gaining popularity with parents, who record their child's sleep patterns on a daily basis, making this assessment tool even more accessible.[19] Objective sleep assessment may also be useful, given that parent and child reports are subjected to recall bias, especially with regard to nighttime events, some of which parents may not be aware of.[20] Actigraphy and other wearable devices are increasingly used in clinical settings to gauge sleep-wake patterns in youth.[21] Technological advances have also made nearable devices highly accessible. For example, auto-videosomnography is based on computer-vision technology, wherein an algorithm translates a child's videoed motion-stillness patterns (recorded using camera baby monitors) into sleep-wake patterns.[22,23] Finally, polysomnography (PSG) may be warranted when there are indications of respiratory issues (eg, loud snoring, gasping) or restless sleep (eg, frequent kicking movements), requiring differential diagnosis.[24]

Assessment and diagnosis of insomnia pose unique challenges for different developmental stages. Infants and toddlers clearly cannot report on any distress or impairment, thus seeking assessment and treatment depends entirely on caregivers. Given that sleep in the early stages of life is typically fragmented due to the immature physiology governing sleep (ie, the homeostatic and circadian processes),[25] it has been argued that the classification of infant sleep difficulties as insomnia discounts the normal biological developmental progression of sleep and serves twenty-first century western industrialized lifestyles, rather than infants themselves.[26,27] Infant insomnia symptoms may be adverse primarily for parents, posing the question of whether diagnosis is called for, and if so, is it the infant, the parent, or the dyadic/family system that should be diagnosed? Caregivers are usually the ones deciding whether or not to seek assessment and treatment of older children's insomnia symptoms as well. Children may not perceive their sleep as a problem or desire treatment, especially when the latter entails relinquishing parent accommodation (eg, co-sleeping) or avoidance behaviors (eg, school truancy). Assessment complexities also occur in adolescence, as circadian phase delays may account for difficulties initiating sleep (ie, sleep-onset latencies). Early school start times may preclude adequate sleep opportunities, which are required for diagnosis, thus making it difficult to identify the source of the adolescent's sleep issues.[28] Therefore, in more complex cases, integration of both the child and caregivers' perspectives, attainable objective metrics (eg, actigraphic sleep-wake patterns), and possibly feedback from the child's broader environment (eg, the school system) may facilitate diagnosis and allow the development of an appropriate agreed-on treatment plan.

CONSEQUENCES

Insomnia in youth is associated with a myriad of maladaptive consequences. Classification systems list a broad array of impairments as part of the diagnostic criteria, including adverse impact on cognitive (eg, attention, memory), motor (eg, proneness for accidents), emotional (eg, mood, reduced motivation), behavioral (eg, hyperactivity, aggression), and social functioning.[7,8] Correspondingly, cross-sectional research has demonstrated strong links between pediatric insomnia and impairments in executive functions, risk-taking behaviors, poor academic performance, internalizing and externalizing symptoms, obesity, and other poor health outcomes.[28–30] These links are likely complex and bidirectional, with sleep difficulties both driving and being driven by impairments in other domains. When examining the pathway of insomnia's impact on other areas, longitudinal and experimental studies provide convincing evidence for detrimental effects. Longitudinal investigations have indicated that insomnia symptoms in youth predict the onset of internalizing and externalizing disorders, substance abuse, and poor academic performance.[31–33] In a community-based longitudinal study conducted over 7 years from school-age to adolescence, persistent insomnia was associated not only with worse psychosocial quality of life but also with increased risk of developing a chronic medical condition or reporting a new medication.[12] Importantly, evidence suggests that insomnia symptoms are more likely to precede the development of anxiety and depression, rather than the other way around.[31] Experimental manipulations significantly restricting or fragmenting sleep in youth are scarce, partly due to ethical constraints. Still, such studies have demonstrated compromised neurobehavioral and affective functioning following restricted sleep in infants,[34] children,[35,36] and adolescents.[37,38]

It is important to note that pediatric insomnia may be detrimental not only for the young person but also for their family members. Adverse impact has been extensively documented in parents of infants and toddlers. Given the strong dependency on parents early on in development, young children's insomnia symptoms are usually associated with considerable sleep loss for parents, which may result in increased depression, anxiety, stress, poor physical health, and reduced quality of life.[39–41] Insomnia symptoms have also been shown to be associated with negative caregiving emotions and behaviors[42,43] and in extreme cases, with child neglect, infant shaking, and even filicide.[44] Caregiver or family secondary impacts, such as increased stress and daytime sleepiness, may also be apparent in school-age and adolescent insomnia, given the associated heightened parental accommodating behaviors (eg, co-sleeping), although more research is warranted to estimate the extent of these maladaptive consequences in families of older youth.

CAUSE

An intricate combination of intrinsic and extrinsic factors may set the stage for the onset of pediatric insomnia. Intrinsic predisposing factors include genetically determined vulnerability to sleep difficulties, dysregulated temperament, changes in circadian and sleep homeostatic processes, medical conditions, and neurodevelopmental or psychiatric disorders. In a recent systematic review of risk and protective factors for behavioral sleep problems among preschool- and early school–aged children, "difficult" temperament and older age were identified as established biological risk and protective (respectively) factors for pediatric sleep problems.[45] Previous sleep problems, as well as internalizing and externalizing disorders, were recognized as established psychological predisposing and precipitating factors in this age group. Other intrinsic etiologic factors, such as

genetic influence, were found to have a less established evidence base.

Variations in normal developmental trajectories of the 2 main sleep bioregulatory processes may make some youth more susceptible to insomnia. "Process S" refers to the sleep homeostat, which regulates the sleep drive, accumulating with prolonged periods of wakefulness.[46] "Process C" refers to the endogenous circadian oscillator, which interacts with the sleep homeostat and with external zeitgebers (eg, light signals) to regulate 24-hour sleep propensity. Processes S and C undergo 2 periods of dramatic evolution across development. First, in infancy, homeostatic sleep pressure and circadian rhythms rapidly mature, facilitating the consolidation of polyphasic sleep into a monophasic nocturnal episode.[25] The maturation of these processes, however, may take longer for some infants and toddlers, resulting in increased sleep fragmentation across the 24-hour day. In adolescence, a further "developmental leap" occurs—a reduction in the accumulation of homeostatic sleep pressure, in concert with a delay in circadian phase, prime adolescents for longer sleep-onset latencies and poorer sleep efficiency, and/or later sleep onset times and shorter sleep duration (given that sleep opportunities are often curtailed by school start times).[47] Hence, the normal progression of physiologic processes that govern sleep may be implicated in the emergence of insomnia symptoms in infancy and in adolescence.

Research into the pathogenesis of insomnia suggests that hyperarousal is also a key contributor.[28] The hyperarousal model, originally developed to describe adult insomnia pathophysiology, posits that elevated levels of cortical arousal, somatic processes (eg, metabolism, inflammation), and cognitive activity (eg, racing thoughts), interacting with other predisposing, precipitating, and perpetuating factors, underlie insomnia symptomology.[48] Hyperarousal and/or hypoactive sleep-inducing processes are thought to increase sensory processing, thus preventing individuals from falling and/or staying asleep. Although evidence for this model in the adult insomnia literature is abundant, pediatric investigations of hyperarousal in insomnia are scarce. Still, cortical hyperarousal during sleep onset and nonrapid eye movement, as well as elevated inflammation, and hyperaroused cardiac autonomic modulation have been demonstrated in adolescents with insomnia compared with controls.[49–51] Cognitive hyperarousal has additionally been associated with insomnia in youth, typically manifested in older children as rumination and racing thoughts[52] and in younger children as intense nighttime fears or nightmares.[53] Emerging evidence thus suggests that hyperarousal plays a role in causing pediatric insomnia, yet more longitudinal research is warranted to examine these mechanistic pathways across childhood and adolescence.

In a complex interplay with intrinsic influences, extrinsic factors may also shape the onset and perseverance of insomnia in youth. These include environmental, social, and behavioral aspects, often profusely mediated by caregivers, particularly in the earlier stages of development. Newton and colleagues[45] identified increased parental involvement in the child's sleep context as an established risk factor for preschool- and younger school–aged children's behavioral sleep problems. Negative parenting style was additionally indexed as an established caregiver-related risk factor, whereas parental psychopathology and marital conflict were indexed as "emerging" risk factors, with less research evidence to support their role in insomnia development. Adolescent insomnia has also been associated with parent factors, such as parental divorce, adverse parenting styles, and family stress.[52] Still, this evidence is based mostly on cross-sectional studies, and thus further work is needed to examine caregivers' role in adolescent insomnia.

Several additional factors may be implicated in the advent and maintenance of insomnia symptoms. Lower socioeconomic background and ethnicity/minority status have been recognized as substantial risk factors in both children and adolescents.[45,54] Media screen exposure and use have also been proposed as precipitating factors for the development of insomnia.[55,56] Although most of the research in this domain has focused on adolescents, emerging evidence indicates that digital screen exposure may also be displacing sleep in young children and even in infants.[57,58] Other risk factors are applicable mostly to adolescents. Increased caffeine and alcohol intake may lead to difficulties initiating or maintaining sleep.[59,60] Social and academic responsibilities (eg, friendships, school work, participation in competitive sports) also tend to increase in adolescence, often inducing insomnia symptoms either by restricting sleep opportunities or by generating elevated stress and hyperarousal.[28]

TREATMENT

Cognitive behavior approaches are considered as the first-line treatment of insomnia in youth.[10] These interventions are often based on learning theory and target child and/or parent behaviors and cognitions to address fragmented or insufficient sleep. They include a broad spectrum of techniques, sometimes "packaged" as cognitive-behavior therapy for insomnia (CBT-I). Systematic reviews and meta-analyses have consistently demonstrated the benefits of these treatment approaches in children[61,62] as well as adolescents.[63] In their recent scoping review of 120 studies evaluating behavioral treatments for pediatric insomnia, Meltzer and colleagues[64] found moderate to strong empirical evidence of efficacy.

The main cognitive and behavioral approaches used to treat insomnia in youth include psychoeducation, sleep-promoting bedtime routines and sleep hygiene, stimulus control, sleep restriction, exposure or extinction, reinforcement management, cognitive restructuring, relaxation techniques, and mindfulness. Psychoeducation is often used as a low-intensity, low-cost prevention strategy or first-step approach to address mild cases of insomnia.[64,65] For more severe cases, it is usually the first treatment module administered, setting the stage for subsequent more intense modules (eg, exposure). Psychoeducation may cover a broad range of topics, depending on the child's age and symptoms. These topics include typical sleep development and recommended durations, circadian rhythms, sleep homeostatic pressure, sleep architecture, constructive sleep associations, and parental involvement in the sleep context.

Promoting positive bedtime routines, regulating sleep-context stimuli, and practicing good sleep hygiene are also ubiquitous treatment approaches for insomnia. In early childhood, recommended bedtime routines entail a consistent sequence of 2 to 4 activities, such as bathing and reading stories, lasting no longer than 40 mins, performed calmly, in dim-light conditions, and followed by lights out.[66] These routines aim to strengthen associations between sleep-promoting stimuli and sleep onset, increase predictability of sleep schedules, and thus regulate not only behavioral and emotional responses to the sleep context but also the child's circadian rhythms, provided that bedtimes are consistent across nights. Sleep hygiene similarly addresses stimuli that may hinder or promote sleep but refers to a broader time frame—beyond the hour leading up to sleep onset. For example, sleep hygiene recommendations include avoiding daytime naps, caffeine and alcohol intake, and excessive sedentary time, as well as ensuring optimal conditions for sleep (eg, a dark, cool, quiet, screen-free bedroom).[67] Correspondingly, stimulus control therapy techniques are intended at facilitating sleep onset by separating stimuli associated with sleep (eg, the bed) from those associated with other activities (eg, watching TV).[68] Instructions suggest going to sleep when sleepy, avoiding activities other than sleep in the bedroom as much as possible, and leaving the bedroom if unable to fall asleep.

Although psychoeducation, bedtime routines, sleep hygiene, and stimulus control approaches provide an important foundation for addressing sleep difficulties in youth, they may not always be sufficient for more severe cases of insomnia. Sleep restriction therapy is a more intensive treatment strategy, in which time in bed is curtailed to match the individual's baseline average true sleep time.[69] This restricted and consistent sleep schedule is intended to regularize and entrain circadian rhythms and assure that homeostatic sleep pressure is sufficiently elevated when sleep is attempted so that time in bed is mostly spent asleep rather than awake. Consequently, the bed and bedroom environment become more closely associated with feeling sleepy and falling asleep. A similar approach, developed for young children, is called "bedtime fading." Here, the sleep window is first restricted by delaying bedtimes and then titrated by "fading" bedtimes earlier by 15 minutes at a time.[70] In contrast to the increasing recognition and popularity of sleep restriction in the treatment of adult insomnia, this approach is less frequently used for treating insomnia in youth.[64] In adolescents, this may be due to the typical sleep restriction already apparent, given late bedtimes and early school start times.[47] Further curtailment of sleep may thus beget extremely short sleep durations and exacerbate daytime consequences. Yet, in infants, preschool, and school-aged children, particularly those portraying bedtime resistance, sleep restriction, or bedtime fading may have considerable advantages. These approaches are more gentle and easier to implement compared with graduated extinction or cognitive approaches. Child distress and bedtime conflicts could be dampened by increased child sleepiness when lights out time is delayed. Moreover, these approaches tend to elicit child motivation, due to the appeal of having a later bedtime. Hence, they can facilitate extinction protocols, which the child may embark with both higher motivation and elevated sleep pressure. Recent work has correspondingly demonstrated the benefits of sleep restriction or bedtime fading in young children with insomnia,[71–73] yet additional research is needed to establish their efficacy in pediatric populations.

Extinction or exposure therapy strategies have been shown to be highly efficacious for insomnia in children, particularly those with nighttime fears, bedtime avoidance or refusal, and/or high reliance on parents for regulation in the sleep context. These strategies promote self-regulation by reducing parent involvement and exposing the child to the challenging or fear-provoking situation of attempting sleep independently. As the child learns that they are able to better cope with bedtime on their own, anxiety levels decline, and sleep initiation becomes easier. In infants, such interventions are often termed "sleep training." Several variations exist, including the more intense "unmodified extinction" ("cry it out"), in which parents put the infant to bed drowsy but awake at a set bedtime and then refrain from intervening until a set morning wake-up time.[74] Modified extinction (also called "the Ferber method" or "controlled crying") is a more gradual approach, in which instead of delaying their response throughout the entire night, parents wait for a few minutes before briefly checking-in on their infant for as long as the crying or distress continue.[75] These approaches can be implemented with parental presence (eg, "camping out"), as parents stay next to their child throughout the night, often feigning sleep and delaying their responses to infant distress.[76] In preschool and school-aged children, a graduated exposure hierarchy can be planned, with each step introducing greater child independence (eg, reducing parent proximity at bedtime by moving the parent's position farther away from the child's bed or reducing the frequency of parental checking-in visits).[77] Reinforcement management (eg, sticker reward charts) may increase child motivation to follow through with targeted goals and gradually advance through the exposure hierarchy.

Whereas insomnia in younger children is often best targeted by behavioral strategies, more sophisticated cognitive approaches could be used for older youth. Cognitive restructuring, challenging negative sleep-related beliefs or catastrophizing thoughts (eg, "I will never be able to fall asleep," "there is a robber in our backyard"), and rehearsing alternative thoughts (eg, "I will fall asleep eventually," "It might be the wind or a cat in our backyard") have been successfully used to treat insomnia in school-aged children and adolescents.[63,77,78] CBT-I protocols for older youth may also include relaxation techniques, such as breathing exercises, body scans, and progressive muscle relaxation. These techniques could be integrated with mindfulness practices to reduce bedtime stress, anxiety, and hyperarousal.[79,80]

Although evidence for the efficacy of cognitive behavior sleep interventions for pediatric insomnia is mounting, considerable challenges still remain. Several large-scale randomized controlled trials have been conducted in infant and adolescent populations, whereas school-aged children have received limited research attention.[64] Moreover, although ample studies have evaluated CBT-I for children with neurodevelopmental disorders (mostly autism and ADHD), there is a dearth of studies focusing on youth with other psychiatric or medical concerns. In addition, most of the studies have been conducted in Westernized countries with Caucasian youth. High-quality trials are thus warranted to evaluate cognitive and behavioral interventions within more diverse samples around the world. Increasing accessibility and adherence to these treatments is another substantial challenge. Group and digitalized formats of CBT-I have yielded promising results,[19,81] and these cost-effective alternative delivery methods could be particularly suited for adolescents, who may be more concerned about stigmatization. Furthermore, attempts to identify predictors and moderators of treatment outcomes in this field are currently only in their infancy,[82–84] and future efforts in this direction may optimize therapeutic acceptability and cost-effectiveness. A further issue pertains to the limited understanding of mechanistic pathways by which certain treatment components exercise their benefits. Most studies have used a combination of treatment modules, thus not allowing evaluation of individual components. Dismantling studies, "microrandomized trials," and examination of mediation effects could shed light on the underlying mechanisms of these treatments. Initial efforts in this direction have shown, for example, that improvements in bedtime hyperarousal—but not in sleep-hygiene awareness—led to improved sleep quality following a CBT and mindfulness intervention in adolescents.[80] Similar research endeavors could be attempted to understand whether circadian alignment, hyperarousal, sleep architecture, and child or parent cognitions or behavior mediate the impact of specific therapeutic components. Finally, future research should aim to examine the long-term effects of these interventions on sleep as well as other child and parent well-being outcomes. de Bruin and colleagues[85] demonstrated reductions not only in insomnia symptoms but also in psychopathology, following CBT-I for adolescents. Importantly, improvements in sleep mediated the effects on mood, anxiety, and ADHD. Targeting insomnia may be a promising first-step intervention for youth with comorbid anxiety or depression, given that acceptability and adherence may be higher when sleep—rather than emotions—is the initial focus of treatment.[86]

Pharmacologic interventions are also used to treat insomnia in youth, either in isolation or in combination with cognitive behavior interventions.

Predominantly, the use of exogenous melatonin in the treatment of pediatric sleep problems has greatly increased over the past 2 decades. This synthetic hormone can reduce sleep-onset latency (when delivered in immediate-release form) and increase sleep consolidation (when delivered in prolonged-release form). In a meta-analysis of 7 trials across 387 children and adolescents with insomnia, exogenous melatonin was found to be superior to placebo in reducing sleep-onset latency and increasing total sleep time.[87] Although concerns have been raised regarding the safety of exogeneous melatonin use in youth, this meta-analysis revealed little to no difference in short-term side effects of melatonin compared with placebo. Still, more studies are needed to evaluate the safety of this treatment in the long term. Other medications, such as sedating antihistamines, benzodiazepines, antidepressants, α2-receptor agonists, pyrimidine derivatives, and antipsychotics, are also sometimes prescribed for children and adolescents with insomnia. These pharmacologic interventions are most commonly used for youth with comorbid medical, psychiatric, and/or neurodevelopmental conditions.[88,89] However, neither melatonin nor any of these drugs have been approved by the US Food and Drug Administration, and only prolonged-release melatonin has been approved by the European Medicines Agency for the treatment of pediatric insomnia. Given the ubiquitous "off-label" prescription of these medications, and high accessibility of melatonin either over-the-counter or online, more work is needed to inform regulation and ensure the safe and effective use of pharmacotherapy in youth with insomnia.

SUMMARY

Insomnia disorder in youth is highly prevalent and associated with a myriad of maladaptive consequences for the child and family, yet remains largely underdiagnosed. It is thus strongly recommended that medical and psychiatric evaluations of youth routinely include assessment of sleep-wake patterns. Diagnosis can be determined based on a clinical interview in most cases, although sleep diaries and objective sleep assessment can be helpful, particularly when differential diagnosis of other sleep disorders is warranted. Although several intrinsic and extrinsic risk factors for pediatric insomnia have been identified, the pathophysiology of this disorder remains largely unknown. Evidence of hyperarousal as an underlying mechanism has begun to emerge, particularly in adolescents, yet future work is needed to explore the neurophysiology of insomnia in early life. Cognitive behavior therapy techniques have received substantial empirical support in pediatric populations. Still, future work should aim to assess these interventions in school-aged children as well as in more diverse populations; increase their accessibility; identify predictors, moderators, and mediators of treatment outcomes; and assess their long-term effects on sleep and mental health. Additional research is also warranted to evaluate the efficacy and safety of pharmacotherapy for pediatric insomnia. Efforts to broaden our understanding of insomnia early on in life are crucial for optimizing care, minimizing the adverse consequences of this disorder, and possibly preventing its persistence into adulthood.

CLINICS CARE POINTS

- Assessment of sleep-wake patterns should be routinely included in any medical or psychiatric evaluation of infants, children, and adolescents.

- Diagnosis of insomnia can generally be based on a clinical interview with the child and/or caregivers, taking into account the child's broad developmental, environmental, and behavioral context.

- Objective sleep assessment (eg, via actigraphy, PSG, or auto-videosomnography) can be useful for differential diagnosis and characterizing specific clinical features.

- Cognitive behavior interventions are considered the first-line treatment of insomnia in youth, with sound evidence for efficacy and safety.

- Pharmacotherapy, and especially exogeneous melatonin, is frequently used for pediatric insomnia, despite the absence of sufficient empirical evidence and regulation. Further investigations into the efficacy and safety of these treatments are thus essential to inform regulatory guidelines and ensure adequate practice.

DISCLOSURE

The author has no conflicting interests to disclose.

REFERENCES

1. Hirshkowitz M, Whiton K, Albert SM, et al. National Sleep Foundation's sleep time duration recommendations: methodology and results summary. Sleep health 2015; 1(1):40–3.

2. Sadeh A, Tikotzky L, Kahn M. Sleep in infancy and childhood: implications for emotional and behavioral difficulties in adolescence and beyond. Curr Opin Psychiatry 2014;27(6):453–9.

3. Spruyt K. A review of developmental consequences of poor sleep in childhood. Sleep Med 2019;60: 3–12.

4. Meltzer LJ, Johnson C, Crosette J, et al. Prevalence of diagnosed sleep disorders in pediatric primary care practices. Pediatrics 2010;125(6):e1410–8.

5. Fernandez-Mendoza J, Lenker KP, Calhoun SL, et al. Trajectories of insomnia symptoms from childhood through young adulthood. Pediatrics 2022; 149(3). e2021053616.

6. American Academy of Sleep Medicine. International classification of sleep disorders (ICSD-2). Diagnostic and coding manual. 2005.

7. American Academy of Sleep Medicine, The international classification of sleep disorders:(ICSD-3), 2014, American Academy of Sleep Medicine Darien, IL.

8. American Psychiatric Association. Diagnostic and statistical manual of mental disorders (DSM-5®). Arlington, VA: American Psychiatric Pub; 2013.

9. Edinger JD, Wyatt JK, Stepanski EJ, et al. Testing the reliability and validity of DSM-IV-TR and ICSD-2 insomnia diagnoses: results of a multitrait-multimethod analysis. Arch Gen Psychiatry 2011; 68(10):992–1002.

10. Medalie L, Dang T, Casnar CL. Pediatric insomnia: etiology, impact, assessment, and treatment. Pediatric sleep medicine. Cham: Springer, Springer; 2021. p. 333–9.

11. Johnson EO, Roth T, Schultz L, et al. Epidemiology of DSM-IV insomnia in adolescence: lifetime prevalence, chronicity, and an emergent gender difference. Pediatrics 2006;117(2):e247–56.

12. Combs D, Goodwin JL, Quan SF, et al. Insomnia, health-related quality of life and health outcomes in children: a seven year longitudinal cohort. Sci Rep 2016;6(1):1–10.

13. Shelton AR, Malow B. Neurodevelopmental disorders commonly presenting with sleep disturbances. Neurotherapeutics 2021;18(1):156–69.

14. Souders MC, Zavodny S, Eriksen W, et al. Sleep in children with autism spectrum disorder. Curr Psychiatr Rep 2017;19(6):1–17.

15. Mindell JA, Sadeh A, Kwon R, et al. Cross-cultural differences in the sleep of preschool children. Sleep Med 2013;14(12):1283–9.

16. Sadeh A. A brief screening questionnaire for infant sleep problems: validation and findings for an Internet sample. Pediatrics 2004;113(6):1795.

17. Owens JA, Spirito A, McGuinn M. The Children's Sleep Habits Questionnaire (CSHQ): psychometric

properties of a survey instrument for school-aged children. Sleep-New York- 2000;23(8):1043–52.

18. Morin CM, Belleville G, Bélanger L, et al. The Insomnia Severity Index: psychometric indicators to detect insomnia cases and evaluate treatment response. Sleep 2011;34(5):601–8.

19. Schlarb AA, Kater M-J, Werner A, et al. Sleep apps for children—a critical view. Somnologie 2021;25(1):4–10.

20. Sadeh A. Sleep assessment methods. Monogr Soc Res Child Dev 2015;80(1):33–48.

21. Schoch SF, Kurth S, Werner H. Actigraphy in sleep research with infants and young children: current practices and future benefits of standardized reporting. J Sleep Res 2021;30(3):e13134.

22. Kahn M, Barnett N, Glazer A, et al. COVID-19 babies: auto-videosomnography and parent reports of infant sleep, screen time, and parent well-being in 2019 vs 2020. Sleep Med 2021;85:259–67.

23. Kahn M, Gradisar M. Sleeping through COVID-19: a longitudinal comparison of 2019 and 2020 infant auto-videosomnography metrics. J Child Psychol Psychiatry 2021;63(6):693–700.

24. Bruni O, DelRosso L, Mogavero MP, et al. Is behavioral insomnia "purely behavioral". J Clin Sleep Med 2022;18(5):1475–6.

25. Jenni OG, LeBourgeois MK. Understanding sleep–wake behavior and sleep disorders in children: the value of a model. Curr Opin Psychiatry 2006;19(3):282.

26. Blunden SL, Thompson KR, Dawson D. Behavioural sleep treatments and night time crying in infants: challenging the status quo. Sleep Med Rev 2011;15(5):327–34.

27. Ball HL, Tomori C, McKenna JJ. Toward an integrated anthropology of infant sleep. AA 2019;121(3):595–612.

28. de Zambotti M, Goldstone A, Colrain IM, et al. Insomnia disorder in adolescence: diagnosis, impact, and treatment. Sleep Med Rev 2018;39:12–24.

29. Bruni O, Melegari MG, Esposito A, et al. Executive functions in preschool children with chronic insomnia. J Clin Sleep Med 2020;16(2):231–41.

30. Zhao K, Zhang J, Wu Z, et al. The relationship between insomnia symptoms and school performance among 4966 adolescents in Shanghai, China. Sleep Health 2019;5(3):273–9.

31. Lovato N, Gradisar M. A meta-analysis and model of the relationship between sleep and depression in adolescents: recommendations for future research and clinical practice. Sleep Med Rev 2014;18(6):521–9.

32. Mike TB, Shaw DS, Forbes EE, et al. The hazards of bad sleep—sleep duration and quality as predictors of adolescent alcohol and cannabis use. Drug Alcohol Depend 2016;168:335–9.

33. Zhang L, Yang Y, Luo Y, et al. A longitudinal study of insomnia, daytime sleepiness, and academic performance in Chinese adolescents. Behav Sleep Med 2022;20(6):798–808.

34. Berger RH, Miller AL, Seifer R, et al. Acute sleep restriction effects on emotion responses in 30-to 36-month-old children. J Sleep Res 2012;21(3):235–46.

35. Sadeh A, Gruber R, Raviv A. The effects of sleep restriction and extension on school-age children: what a difference an hour makes. Child Dev 2003;74(2):444–55.

36. Fallone G, Acebo C, Seifer R, et al. Experimental restriction of sleep opportunity in children: effects on teacher ratings. Sleep 2005;28(12):1561–7.

37. Baum KT, Desai A, Field J, et al. Sleep restriction worsens mood and emotion regulation in adolescents. J Child Psychol Psychiatry 2014;55(2):180–90.

38. McMakin DL, Dahl RE, Buysse DJ, et al. The impact of experimental sleep restriction on affective functioning in social and nonsocial contexts among adolescents. J Child Psychol Psychiatry 2016;57(9):1027–37.

39. Liew SC, Aung T. Sleep deprivation and its association with diseases-a review. Sleep Med 2021;77:192–204.

40. Sadeh A, Tikotzky L, Scher A. Parenting and infant sleep. Sleep Med Rev 2010;14(2):89–96.

41. Bayer JK, Hiscock H, Hampton A, et al. Sleep problems in young infants and maternal mental and physical health. J Paediatr Child Health 2007;43(1-2):66–73.

42. King LS, Rangel E, Simpson N, et al. Mothers' postpartum sleep disturbance is associated with the ability to sustain sensitivity toward infants. Sleep Med 2020;65:74–83.

43. McQuillan ME, Bates JE, Staples AD, et al. Maternal stress, sleep, and parenting. J Fam Psychol 2019;33(3):349.

44. Bartels L, Easteal P. Mothers who kill: the forensic use and judicial reception of evidence of postnatal depression and other psychiatric disorders in Australian filicide cases. Melb Univ Law Rev 2013;37(2):297–341.

45. Newton AT, Honaker SM, Reid GJ. Risk and protective factors and processes for behavioral sleep problems among preschool and early school-aged children: a systematic review. Sleep Med Rev 2020;52:101303.

46. Borbély AA. A two process model of sleep regulation. Hum Neurobiol 1982;1(3):195–204.

47. Crowley SJ, Wolfson AR, Tarokh L, et al. An update on adolescent sleep: new evidence informing the perfect storm model. J Adolesc 2018;67:55–65.

48. Riemann D, Spiegelhalder K, Feige B, et al. The hyperarousal model of insomnia: a review of the concept and its evidence. Sleep Med Rev 2010;14(1):19–31.

49. Fernandez-Mendoza J, Li Y, Vgontzas AN, et al. Insomnia is associated with cortical hyperarousal as early as adolescence. Sleep 2016;39(5):1029–36.

50. Fernandez-Mendoza J, Baker JH, Vgontzas AN, et al. Insomnia symptoms with objective short sleep duration are associated with systemic inflammation in adolescents. Brain Behav Immun 2017;61:110–6.

51. Rodríguez-Colón SM, He F, Bixler EO, et al. Sleep variability and cardiac autonomic modulation in adolescents–Penn State Child Cohort (PSCC) study. Sleep Med 2015;16(1):67–72.

52. Blake MJ, Trinder JA, Allen NB. Mechanisms underlying the association between insomnia, anxiety, and depression in adolescence: implications for behavioral sleep interventions. Clin Psychol Rev 2018;63:25–40.

53. Reynolds KC, Alfano CA. Things that go bump in the night: frequency and predictors of nightmares in anxious and nonanxious children. Behav Sleep Med 2016;14(4):442–56.

54. Guglielmo D, Gazmararian JA, Chung J, et al. Racial/ethnic sleep disparities in US school-aged children and adolescents: a review of the literature. Sleep health 2018;4(1):68–80.

55. Hale L, Li X, Hartstein LE, et al. Media use and sleep in teenagers: what do we know? Curr Sleep Med Rep 2019;5(3):128–34.

56. Bartel KA, Gradisar M, Williamson P. Protective and risk factors for adolescent sleep: a meta-analytic review. Sleep Med Rev 2015;21:72–85.

57. Nathanson AI, Beyens I. The relation between use of mobile electronic devices and bedtime resistance, sleep duration, and daytime sleepiness among preschoolers. Behav Sleep Med 2018;16(2):202–19.

58. Kahn M, Barnett N, Glazer A, et al. Sleep and screen exposure across the beginning of life: deciphering the links using big-data analytics. Sleep 2020;44(3):zsaa158.

59. Owens JA, Mindell J, Baylor A. Effect of energy drink and caffeinated beverage consumption on sleep, mood, and performance in children and adolescents. Nutr Rev 2014;72(suppl_1):65–71.

60. Marmorstein NR. Sleep patterns and problems among early adolescents: associations with alcohol use. Addict Behav 2017;66:13–6.

61. Mindell JA, Kuhn B, Lewin DS, et al. Behavioral treatment of bedtime problems and night wakings in infants and young children. Sleep 2006;29(10):1263–76.

62. Meltzer LJ, Mindell JA. Systematic review and meta-analysis of behavioral interventions for pediatric insomnia. J Pediatr Psychol 2014;39(8):932–48.

63. Blake MJ, Sheeber LB, Youssef GJ, et al. Systematic review and meta-analysis of adolescent cognitive–behavioral sleep interventions. Clin Child Fam Psychol Rev 2017;20(3):227–49.

64. Meltzer LJ, Wainer A, Engstrom E, et al. A scoping review of behavioral treatments for pediatric insomnia. JAMA Netw Open 2019;2(12):e1918061.

65. Hiscock H. An educational intervention for improving infant sleep duration—why won't you sleep, baby? JAMA Netw Open 2019;2(12):e1918061.

66. Mindell JA, Williamson AA. Benefits of a bedtime routine in young children: sleep, development, and beyond. Sleep Med Rev 2018;40:93–108.

67. Lin C-Y, Strong C, Scott AJ, et al. A cluster randomized controlled trial of a theory-based sleep hygiene intervention for adolescents. Sleep 2018;41(11):zsy170.

68. Bootzin RR. Stimulus control treatment for insomnia. Proceedings of the American Psychological Association 1972;7:395–6.

69. Spielman AJ, Saskin P, Thorpy MJ. Treatment of chronic insomnia by restriction of time in bed. Sleep 1987;10(1):45–56.

70. Piazza CC, Fisher WW. Bedtime fading in the treatment of pediatric insomnia. J Behav Ther Exp Psychiatry 1991;22(1):53–6.

71. Gradisar M, Jackson K, Spurrier NJ, et al. Behavioral interventions for infant sleep problems: a randomized controlled trial. Pediatrics 2016;137(6):e20151486.

72. Cooney MR, Short MA, Gradisar M. An open trial of bedtime fading for sleep disturbances in preschool children: a parent group education approach. Sleep Med 2018;46:98–106.

73. Delemere E, Dounavi K. Parent-implemented bedtime fading and positive routines for children with autism spectrum disorders. J Autism Dev Disord 2018;48(4):1002–19.

74. Rickert VI, Johnson CM. Reducing nocturnal awakening and crying episodes in infants and young children: a comparison between scheduled awakenings and systematic ignoring. Pediatrics 1988;81(2):203–12.

75. Ferber R. Solve your child's sleep problems. New York: Simon & Schuster; 1985.

76. Sadeh A. Assessment of interventions for infant night waking- parental reports and activity-based home monitoring. J Consult Clin Psychol 1994;62(1):63–8.

77. Schlarb AA, Bihlmaier I, Velten-Schurian K, et al. Short-and long-term effects of CBT-I in groups for school-age children suffering from chronic insomnia: the KiSS-program. Behav Sleep Med 2018;16(4):380–97.

78. Paine S, Gradisar M. A randomised controlled trial of cognitive-behaviour therapy for behavioural insomnia of childhood in school-aged children. Behav Res Ther 2011;49(6–7):379–88.

79. de Bruin EJ, Meijer A, Bögels SM. The contribution of a body scan mindfulness meditation to

effectiveness of internet-delivered CBT for insomnia in adolescents. Mindfulness 2020;11(4):872–82.

80. Blake M, Schwartz O, Waloszek JM, et al. The SENSE study: treatment mechanisms of a cognitive behavioral and mindfulness-based group sleep improvement intervention for at-risk adolescents, *Sleep*, 40 (6), 2017, zsx061.

81. McLay L, Sutherland D, Machalicek W, et al. Systematic review of telehealth interventions for the treatment of sleep problems in children and adolescents. J Behav Educ 2020;29(2):222–45.

82. Kahn M, Juda-Hanael M, Livne-Karp E, et al. Behavioral interventions for pediatric insomnia: one treatment may not fit all. Sleep 2019;43(4):zsz268.

83. Kahn M, Livne-Karp E, Juda-Hanael M, et al. Behavioral interventions for infant sleep problems: the role of parental cry tolerance and sleep-related cognitions. J Clin Sleep Med 2020;16(8):1275–83.

84. Blake MJ, Blake LM, Schwartz O, et al. Who benefits from adolescent sleep interventions? Moderators of treatment efficacy in a randomized controlled trial of a cognitive-behavioral and mindfulness-based group sleep intervention for at-risk adolescents. J Child Psychol Psychiatry 2018;59(6):637–49.

85. de Bruin EJ, Bögels SM, Oort FJ, et al. Improvements of adolescent psychopathology after insomnia treatment: results from a randomized controlled trial over 1 year. J Child Psychol Psychiatry 2018;59(5):509–22.

86. Gradisar M, Kahn M, Micic G, et al. Sleep's role in the development and resolution of adolescent depression. Nature Reviews Psychology 2022;1(9):512–23.

87. Wei S, Smits MG, Tang X, et al. Efficacy and safety of melatonin for sleep onset insomnia in children and adolescents: a meta-analysis of randomized controlled trials. Sleep Med 2020;68:1–8.

88. Bruni O, Angriman M, Melegari MG, et al. Pharmacotherapeutic management of sleep disorders in children with neurodevelopmental disorders. Expert Opin Pharmacother 2019;20(18):2257–71.

89. Barrett JR, Tracy DK, Giaroli G. To sleep or not to sleep: a systematic review of the literature of pharmacological treatments of insomnia in children and adolescents with attention-deficit/hyperactivity disorder. J Child Adolesc Psychopharmacol 2013;23(10):640–7.

Beyond Polysomnography
Clinical Assessment of Pediatric Sleep Health and Sleep Problems

Lisa J. Meltzer, PhD[a,b,*], Courtney Paisley, PhD[b,c]

KEYWORDS

- Infant • Toddler • Preschooler • School-aged • Adolescent • Patient-reported outcomes
- Questionnaires

KEY POINTS

- Pediatric sleep health and sleep problems should be viewed from a developmental, socioecological framework.
- Child self-report of sleep health and sleep problems should be included in clinical assessments when developmentally appropriate, typically starting around the age of 8 years.
- Screening for pediatric sleep health and sleep problems should be part of every routine primary care visit and should be included in standard assessments in specialty care clinics.
- Prospective sleep diaries provide a wealth of information about a child's typical sleep-wake patterns, assisting with differential diagnoses and treatment planning.
- Validated, subjective questionnaires can be used both for screening and to monitor progress with treatment recommendations.

Sleep is ubiquitous for pediatric patients and is integral for every aspect of health and well-being. As sleep needs and sleep patterns change across development, it is essential to understand both sleep health and sleep problems in a clinical setting. This chapter reviews the clinical assessment of pediatric sleep health and pediatric sleep problems, with strategies and tools that can be integrated into both primary care and specialty care practice.

PEDIATRIC SLEEP HEALTH

Pediatric sleep health has been defined as "subjective or caregiver-rated satisfaction, appropriate timing, adequate duration for age, high efficiency, sustained alertness during waking hours, and healthy sleep behaviors" (p.7).[1] Per the definition, there are 6 dimensions of pediatric sleep that should be considered in clinical assessment, with

the acronym Peds B-SATED used as a guide. In *Pediatrics*, these dimensions are sleep-related *Be*haviors, *S*atisfaction with sleep, *A*lertness during waking hours, *T*iming of sleep, sleep *E*fficiency, and sleep *D*uration. Each of these dimensions will be considered in the discussion of clinical assessment later in this chapter.

Focusing on the positive attributes of sleep health, rather than exclusively on sleep disorders, allows for health promotion and prevention. The need to distinguish pediatric versus adult sleep health is also important, as children live within a complex socioecological system that has a direct and indirect impact on child sleep.[1–3] Understanding pediatric sleep within this system guides assessment and treatment. For example, individual factors such as age and chronotype have a significant impact on the *timing* and *duration* of pediatric sleep, whereas genetics and health comorbidities may affect sleep *efficiency* and

[a] National Jewish Health, 1400 Jackson Street, G322, Denver, CO 80206, USA; [b] University of Colorado Denver, Anschutz Medical Campus; [c] Children's Hospital Colorado, Developmental Pediatrics, 13123 East 16th Avenue, Box B140, Aurora, CO 80045, USA
* Corresponding author. 1400 Jackson Street, G322, Denver, CO 80206.
E-mail address: meltzerL@njhealth.org

Sleep Med Clin 18 (2023) 147–160
https://doi.org/10.1016/j.jsmc.2023.02.001
1556-407X/23/© 2023 Elsevier Inc. All rights reserved.

alertness during waking hours. Family factors, for example, cultural beliefs or parent work schedules, may influence sleep-related *behaviors* and sleep *timing*, whereas school factors, in particular school start times, directly affect sleep *timing* and *duration*. Finally, neighborhood and broader sociocultural factors, including environmental light, noise, and allergens, experiences of racism and discrimination, and/or neighborhood and community violence, may affect sleep-related *behaviors*, sleep *efficiency*, and *satisfaction* with sleep.

PEDIATRIC SLEEP PROBLEMS

Although pediatric sleep should be assessed as a vital sign at all well-child visits, and tracked across development,[4] it is also important to consider sleep problems reported by parents or caregivers (hereafter referred to as parents) or by patients themselves. Sleep problems broadly include general complaints of poor-quality sleep, insufficient sleep, or daytime sleepiness, as well as formal sleep disorders (ie, sleep apnea, narcolepsy, restless legs syndrome, periodic limb movements in sleep, parasomnias, and insomnia).[5]

In the general population, sleep problems have been reported by 11% of early school-aged children (5–6 years) and 7% to 8% of older children/adolescents (8–17 years) and parents.[6,7] Sleep problems are even more common in children/adolescents with allergic disease (47%) and among children/adolescents with autism or children/adolescents who present to a pediatric sleep clinic (up to 90% for both groups).[7,8] A recent international study of young children (ages 0–36 months) found that 35% of parents reported their child had a "sleep problem," whereas 96% identified at least one thing about their child's sleep that they would like to change (eg, bedtime/falling asleep, overnight sleep, morning waking, and naps).[9] Of note, 75% of parents endorsed changes in 3 or more categories, highlighting the significant dissatisfaction with their child's sleep. Thus, it is critical for pediatric health care providers in both primary and specialty care settings to screen for sleep problems.

CLINICAL ASSESSMENT OF PEDIATRIC SLEEP HEALTH AND SLEEP PROBLEMS

The clinical assessment of pediatric sleep can include both subjective and objective assessments.[10] With the focus on pediatric sleep health and sleep problems, this chapter reviews different types of subjective assessments, including a clinical interview, sleep diaries, and questionnaires. Although certain sleep disorders (eg, sleep-

disordered breathing, narcolepsy, periodic limb movements in sleep) can only be diagnosed in a sleep laboratory that includes overnight polysomnography (PSG) and daytime multiple sleep latency testing,[11] and actigraphy is useful for objectively assessing sleep-wake patterns for 1 to 2 weeks in the patient's natural sleep environment,[12] these objective assessments are beyond the scope of this chapter.

Developmental Considerations for Pediatric Sleep Assessment

Unlike adult sleep, pediatric sleep undergoes a number of changes and transitions over the first 18 years of life due to physiologic growth and neurologic development.[13,14] In addition, family, social, and broader environment factors are also changing.[15] Thus, when approaching clinical assessment, it is essential to concurrently consider developmental changes and the dimensions of pediatric sleep health and sleep problems. In addition, it is important to understand when it is appropriate to ask children directly about their sleep rather than relying solely on parental report.

This section reviews the different developmental changes for each sleep health domain, as well as factors that contribute to whether children are able to report on their own sleep health.

Behaviors

Sleep-related behaviors include consistent bedtime routines, sleep-onset associations, caffeine intake, and use of electronic devices before bedtime, in bed, and/or during the night.[1,16] Although these behaviors are present across development, sleep problems are more likely to be reported among younger children, in particular inconsistent bedtime routines and parental presence at sleep onset.[17–20] As children progress through school-age and into adolescents, caffeine intake and use of electronic devices increase.[16,21–23]

Children ages 8 years and older should be able to reliably report on most sleep-related behaviors, although many children and families may not be aware of which products contain caffeine unless that is something regularly discussed within the home.[24] Some older preschool and early school-aged children (4–8 years) are able to report on bedtime routines, sleep-onset associations, and the use of electronics at bedtime, although the duration of electronic use is likely not accurate in younger children.

Satisfaction/Quality

As this dimension focuses on the subjective assessment of "good" or "poor" sleep, it is one of the most difficult to quantify,[25] especially in younger children who are unlikely to complain of poor sleep quality/dissatisfaction with sleep. However, it is important to keep in mind that parental report of sleep quality, especially in younger children or in children with neurodevelopmental disorders, may be biased by the parent's own sleep quality. For example, in 2 families a young child wakes the parent during the night. In family A, the parent returns to sleep quickly and feels rested in the morning, thus does not report that the child has poor sleep quality. In family B, the parent is unable to return to sleep and is sleepy the next day and thus reports the child has poor sleep quality. Similarly, studies have shown that parents of children with attention-deficit/hyperactivity disorder (ADHD) report poorer child sleep quality, even though objective measures of sleep do not differ between children with and without ADHD.[26–28] Because of the subjective nature of sleep satisfaction/quality, it is very important to ask older school-aged children and adolescents directly about this aspect of sleep health.

Alertness/Sleepiness

Most younger children are unable to report on or attribute their daytime alertness/sleepiness to nighttime sleep (or naps), so parents should be asked directly about the daytime functioning of young children. That said, it is important to note that many parents may not be aware that young children can become more hyperactive or energetic when sleepy. Thus, it is important to query hyperactivity when screening for daytime alertness/sleepiness. Further, although napping is considered a hallmark of daytime sleepiness in adults, napping is age-appropriate in young children. Although many children stop napping between the ages of 3 and 5 years, approximately 20% of 5-year-old children continue to have a daily nap.[29]

Older children and adolescents (8 years and older) should be directly asked about feelings of alertness/sleepiness, as parent reporters may not always be aware of this subjective experience, unless there are observable behaviors (eg, napping) or reports from the school (eg, child falling asleep in class). Finally, napping in adolescents should be considered within the context of insufficient sleep duration, which is often a result of early school start times.

Timing

The ability to report on the placement of sleep across a 24-hour day relies on a child's ability to tell time. This skill is typically introduced when children start school (around 5 years), and by 8 years, most children should be able to tell time. However, school-aged children may still not be able to report on bedtimes and wake times if parents do not discuss or reinforce this idea (eg, "bedtime is at 8:00 PM, you need to wake up at 7:30 AM for school"). In addition, for younger children who wake spontaneously, wake times may be earlier than reported by parents.

As children get older, the discrepancy increases between parent- and child-reported sleep timing.[30–32] Although there may be a parent-set bedtime for adolescents, and parents are often involved with waking adolescents in the morning, many parents may not be aware of when their adolescent actually attempts to fall asleep; this may be the case especially for parents who go to sleep earlier than their adolescent or who are working in the evenings/overnight.

Efficiency

The ease of falling asleep and returning to sleep is one of the most challenging subjective aspects of sleep health to report, both for children and adults. It is difficult to accurately estimate how long it takes to fall asleep or how long a person is awake during the night. However, older children and adolescents should be asked about sleep-onset latency and night waking frequency/duration, as the perception of these variables are used in the treatment of insomnia. Greater emphasis should be placed on the subjective experience rather than potential objective measures (eg, actigraphy) that likely overestimate sleep due to motionless wakefulness in older children and adolescents (ie, laying still for prolonged periods of time while awake, with devices that use accelerometers to capture sleep-wake patterns incorrectly scoring this as sleep).[33,34]

Duration

Sleep duration includes sleep across the 24-hour window, including during the daytime. As previously stated, expectations for sleep duration change across development, and even within each developmental group there is wide variability in terms of what is considered "normal."[13] In order to report on sleep duration, a child must have a developed sense of time to estimate how many hours they are sleeping; this will not be possible for young children, but even some school-aged children and adolescents may struggle with this concept if they do not have a strong sense of time or ability to calculate time differences from bedtime to wake time. However, it is important to keep in mind that parents of older children and adolescents may also not be able to accurately report sleep duration, as parents become less involved with bedtimes routines and sleep timing (see earlier discussion) as children/adolescents become more independent.

Initial Screening for Sleep Health and Sleep Problems

In the primary care setting, providers should begin with at least 2 screening questions. First, "do you (or your child) have problems sleeping?" Although this question is open to interpretation, it provides patients and parents the opportunity to discuss what they consider to be problematic about sleep, whether it be difficulties falling asleep, waking during the night, waking too early or difficulties waking in the morning, and/or daytime sleepiness. Thus, a positive endorsement to this screening question allows the clinician the opportunity to further query specific areas of sleep.

Second, the American Academy of Pediatrics recommends that all children be screened for snoring (ie, asking parents if their child snores or asking older children/adolescents if their siblings or friends have ever complained that they snore).[35] If positively endorsed, additional questions should ask how frequent and how loud the snoring is and whether the patient is experiencing any issues with daytime alertness/sleepiness. A patient with regular loud snoring should be further evaluated for (or referred for further evaluation of) sleep-disordered breathing.

Simply asking a child (or parent) how much sleep a child gets each night, without the 2 previous questions, is not sufficient. As previously stated, there is a wide range of what is considered "normal" in terms of sleep duration, and sleep duration questions should include both nighttime and daytime sleep. Further, without additional questions about daytime functioning, a single question about duration is not sufficient to identify sleep problems. It is also important to understand the significant night-to-night variability in the sleep of children and adolescents. For example, adolescents will often shift their sleep-wake schedules on weekends (known as social jetlag), as well as significantly increase their sleep duration on weekends (by 2 or more hours) in order to compensate for insufficient sleep duration during the school week.[36]

Detailed Screening for Sleep Health and Sleep Problems

Most general behavioral sleep problems, including insomnia, are related to sleep *timing*, *duration*, and *behaviors*. These 3 areas should be the main focus for primary and specialty care clinicians when conducting a detailed screening. By asking patients/ parents about a typical day, the clinician can begin to identify potential factors contributing to sleep problems.[5]

What time do you have dinner? This question is a good place to start to help families focus on their evening and sleep routines. Consistent routines are essential for good sleep health and can help to prevent sleep problems.[18,37] However, many families do not have a consistent dinner time due to parent work schedules or child extracurricular activities/athletics/employment; this can contribute to irregular evening routines, which in turn can affect sleep onset.

What happens after dinner? This question again helps families to focus on evening activities and bedtime routines, with the clinician able to gather step-by-step information about evening activities (eg, relaxing vs stimulating) and the bedtime routine (including the routine's start time, duration, and consistency). The evening report should end with separate questions about what time the child gets into bed versus what time the child tries to fall asleep. Inconsistent or variable bedtimes can contribute to difficulties with sleep initiation.[38,39] Thus, it is important to ask about routines on weekdays, weekends, and over holidays/summer vacations.

How long does it take you/your child to fall asleep once you turn the light off/try to fall asleep? Is there anything you/your child needs to fall asleep? Difficulty falling asleep is common, but there are many different reasons for prolonged sleep onset, often changing across development. For young children, the second part of this question focuses on sleep onset associations (eg, parent rocking or feeding an infant to sleep, parent lying next to a child to help them fall asleep). However, sleep-onset associations (eg, parents, music, videos) also are present for older children and adolescents.[16,19] Without these associations, sleep onset can be delayed. Even more problematic for many patients/families, if these associations are not present following normal nighttime arousals, children may experience frequent or prolonged night awakenings.[5]

Other factors that may be identified by this question include limit-setting issues (eg, child makes frequent "curtain calls" or requests), child anxiety, or a delayed circadian sleep-wake rhythm. For this last consideration, an additional question can be asked: *If you/your child go to bed later, do you/your child fall asleep faster?* A positive endorsement of this question suggests a faded bedtime treatment approach,[40] whereas a negative endorsement suggests treatment of insomnia or anxiety may be more appropriate.

Once asleep, do you (does your child) wake during the night? If yes, how often, at what time, for how long, and what do you (does your child) do during these awakenings? These questions can again assist with treatment planning. For a child with insomnia, it is important to gain an understanding of what happens following nighttime awakenings (eg, parent rocks child back to sleep, child spends hours worrying about school or not being able to sleep) and whether any electronics devices are used (eg, child turns on the television or watches the clock). However, a child who has a prolonged sleep-onset latency but then sleeps through the night without issue is more likely dealing with a limit-setting or circadian-related sleep problem.

What time do you wake up on school days, weekends, and holidays? Is it difficult to wake up and get going in the morning? The first part of these questions helps to determine sleep opportunity (bedtime to wake time), as well as variability in sleep-wake schedules. When patients or parents report that it is very difficult to wake and start the day, this should be considered alongside the sleep opportunity. Difficulty waking is most commonly a result of insufficient sleep duration. However, patients with sufficient sleep opportunity, but difficulties waking, may need to be further screened for underlying sleep disorders or poor sleep quality.

Does your child nap during the day? Finally, it is important to understand the frequency and duration of daytime napping. Again, for younger children napping is age appropriate and should be considered alongside nighttime sleep when estimating sleep duration.[13] However, in preschool-aged children, the timing and duration of naps may result in delayed sleep onset,[41] which is a common parent-complaint in this age group. School-aged children should typically not be napping, and thus frequent or prolonged naps may be a sign of insufficient sleep duration or poor sleep quality, and further screening for sleep disorders

may be necessary. Adolescents may nap as a way to compensate for insufficient weeknight sleep duration.[36] However, an adolescent who naps, but then still obtains sufficient sleep duration at night, may have an underlying sleep or mood disorder.

Sleep Diaries

Sleep diaries are one of the most useful tools a clinician can use to screen for sleep problems and monitor treatment recommendations. Whenever possible, patients/families should be asked to keep a daily prospective sleep diary before a clinic visit. Sleep diaries can provide a wealth of information about factors that contribute to sleep problems, including sleep timing, duration, and behaviors. A chart type of diary is very useful for this type of screening, providing a snapshot of sleep-wake patterns. By collecting up to 2 weeks of data, the clinician can see variability in night-to-night sleep, as well as other factors that may need to be considered (eg, naps, nighttime behaviors such as nursing a child back to sleep).

Fig. 1 shows a sleep diary for a 10-month-old patient who presented with complaints of frequent night wakings. The diary data show a picture of a consistent bedtime, but inconsistent sleep-onset associations during the night, including nursing, rocking, and bringing the child into the parents' bed.

Fig. 2 is the sleep diary of a 4-year-old who presented with complaints of difficulties falling asleep and prolonged bedtime battles. Data from this diary highlight how the child's nap schedule during the week at preschool was affecting the child's ability to fall asleep at the desired early hour, whereas on weekends when parents would skip the nap, the child was able to fall asleep quickly at the desired earlier bedtime. However, it is important to note that the child obtained the same sleep duration across a 24-hour period,

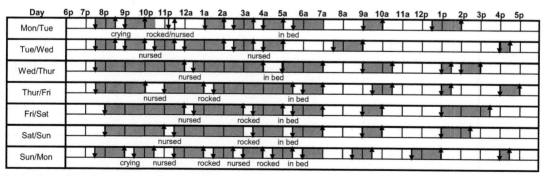

Fig. 1. Sleep diary for a 10-month-old patient who presented with complaints of frequent night wakings, highlighting inconsistent sleep-onset associations.

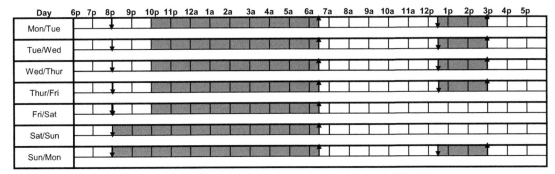

Fig. 2. Sleep diary for a 4-year-old patient who presented with complaints of difficulties falling asleep and prolonged bedtime battles, highlighting the impact of naps on sleep-onset latency.

when both naps and nighttime sleep are considered.

Fig. 3 is the sleep diary of an adolescent who presented with complaints of difficulties sleeping and daytime sleepiness. The data show a picture of insomnia, with difficulties falling asleep and staying asleep, regardless of bedtime. In addition, it is notable that this adolescent was napping during the day, which further perpetuated the insomnia.

Fig. 4 shows the sleep diary of an adolescent who presented with difficulty waking and daytime sleepiness. The data, which included 1 week during school and 1 week during the school break, show a delayed circadian sleep-wake rhythm. It is apparent that when allowed to sleep on their natural biological rhythm, this patient had no difficulties with sleep initiation and maintenance. However, when the sleep-wake schedule was constrained by school start times, this adolescent experienced insufficient sleep duration, resulting in the presenting clinical complaints.

Finally, **Fig. 5** is that of a 9-year-old child who presented due to teacher complaints that the child was falling asleep at school. As this child had a consistent bedtime and wake time, and reportedly no night wakings, further clinical screening was done for underlying sleep disorders, and the parent reported that the child "snored louder than a Mack truck." Thus, the child was referred for an overnight PSG to rule out sleep-disordered breathing.

The Consensus Sleep Diary[42] is another type of prospective diary that provides more detailed data about sleep-wake patterns and is more for cognitive-behavioral therapy for insomnia (CBT-I). Treatment decisions for CBT-I rely heavily on the calculation of sleep efficiency, requiring estimates of time in bed, sleep-onset latency, night waking duration, and total sleep time. The Consensus Sleep Diary provides values that can be used to calculate the necessary values to inform treatment decisions. **Fig. 6** provides graphs of a patient's data before initiation of CBT-I (data were entered into an Excel file for faster calculations and graphing, which helps the adolescent visualize their sleep-wake patterns).

SCREENING QUESTIONNAIRES

A review published in 2020 identified 341 sleep questionnaires[43]; thus a comprehensive review of sleep measures is beyond the scope of this chapter. Instead, the following section will briefly

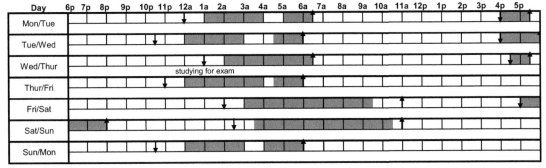

Fig. 3. Sleep diary for an adolescent patient who presented with complaints of difficulties sleeping and daytime sleepiness, with patterns suggestive of insomnia.

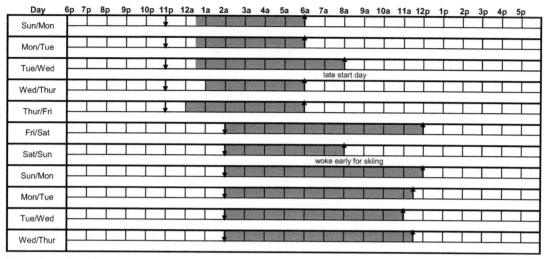

Fig. 4. Sleep diary for an adolescent patient who presented with difficulty waking and daytime sleepiness, with data from 1 week during school and 1 week during school break. Data highlight a delayed circadian sleep-wake rhythm.

discuss (in alphabetical order) commonly used clinical screening measures to assess pediatric sleep health and sleep problems; this will be followed by the presentation of data and case examples for a series of self-report measures for older children and adolescents. When used in combination, these measures can quickly provide patient profiles to guide assessment, differential diagnoses, and treatment of behavioral sleep problems.

The "BEARS" Sleep Screening Tool

The BEARS is a sleep screening tool that provides structured questions to screen for common sleep issues, with parent- and child-reported screening questions modified across developmental age groups.[44] BEARS is an acronym for *B*edtime problems (including difficulty going to bed and falling asleep), *E*xcessive daytime sleepiness, *A*wakenings during the night, *R*egularity of the sleep-

wake schedule and sleep duration, and *S*noring. For each domain there is an initial screening question, and if positively endorsed, a follow-up question asks the parent/patient to describe the problem. When used as a screening tool, the BEARS was found to increase clinician elicited information about sleep problems and specific sleep domains.[44]

Brief Infant Sleep Questionnaire—Revised

The original Brief Infant Sleep Questionnaire (BISQ) was published in 2004 as an 8-item screening measure for children ages 0 to 30 months, including questions about sleep patterns, sleep duration, sleep behaviors, and whether parents believed their child had a sleep problem.[45] Since then, the BISQ has been revised (BISQ-R) and has expanded the assessment age up to 36 months and includes a norm-references

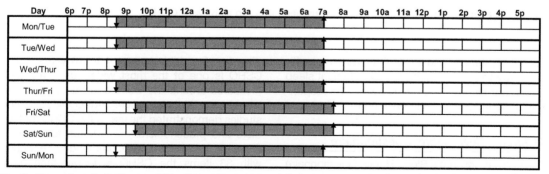

Fig. 5. Sleep diary for a 9-year-old patient who presented due to excessive daytime sleepiness, despite sufficient sleep duration, suggesting an underlying sleep disorder (eg, sleep-disordered breathing).

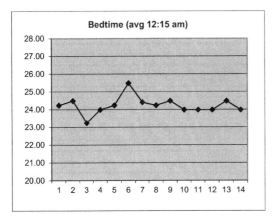

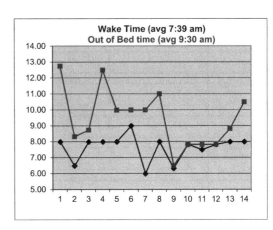

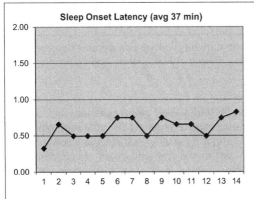

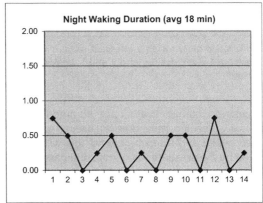

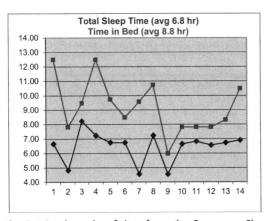

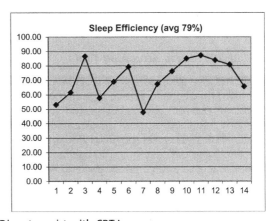

Fig. 6. Visual graphs of data from the Consensus Sleep Diary to assist with CBT-I.

scoring system.[46] The BISQ-R provides an efficient way to collect information about infant sleep before a clinic visit and has shown to be responsive to behavioral sleep interventions.[47,48]

Children's Sleep Habits Questionnaire

The original Children's Sleep Habits Questionnaire (CSHQ) was published in 2000 as a clinical screener of major medical and behavioral sleep disorders for children ages 4 to 10 years.[49] The CSHQ is one of the most widely used research measures around the world and has been translated into multiple languages. Additional validation studies demonstrated the use of the CSHQ for toddlers and preschoolers.[50,51] A cutoff total CSHQ score of 41 has been recommended. Although with 33 items the CSHQ is longer than most screeners, this measure captures all aspects of Peds B-SATED, as well as symptoms of parasomnias and sleep-disordered breathing. A 2017 study validated a modified CSHQ short form (SF-CSHQ), removing the "medically based" items to provide a 23-item screener.[52]

Dysfunctional Beliefs About Sleep

Adapted from the adult version of the Dysfunctional Beliefs and Attitudes about Sleep (DBAS) questionnaire,[53] a 24-item version of the DBAS was initially validated in children ages 8 to 10 years,[54] with a later validated 10-item DBAS for children (DBAS-C10)[55] providing a clinical screener to identify beliefs that may contribute to sleep problems in children and adolescents. Higher scores indicate greater dysfunctional beliefs. Items assess the patient's beliefs about sleep needs, cognitions that interfere with sleep, the short- and long-term consequences of insufficient or poor-quality sleep, and the need to control their sleep. Although there is not a cutoff score, this measure can be quickly scanned by clinicians to identify targeted areas for sleep education and intervention.

Epworth Sleepiness Scale for Children and Adolescents/Modified Epworth Sleepiness Scale

The Epworth Sleepiness Scale (ESS) was developed to assess daytime sleepiness in adults.[56,57] A modified version (mESS) included 8 items that asked parents to report the likelihood that children would fall asleep in different situations. The mESS was first used to assess daytime sleepiness in pediatric patients ages 2 to 18 years with suspected sleep-disordered breathing[58] and was later used in many other studies, including the large CHAT (Childhood Adenotonsillectomy Trial).[59] However, the mESS was not authorized by the copyright holder, and different versions were being used across studies. Thus, the original ESS creator, Dr Murray Johns, developed and validated the Epworth Sleepiness Scale for Children and Adolescents (ESS-CHAD) with 8 age-appropriate items that ask about sleepiness over the past month.[60]

Morningness-Eveningness Scale for Children

The Morningness-Eveningness Scale for Children (M/E) is a 10-item measure that evaluates circadian preference in children and adolescents.[61,62] Lower scores on the M/E indicate an evening preference (a sign of a delayed circadian sleep-wake rhythm). Cutoff scores have been examined, with results indicating the need for different cutoffs based on child age and sex.[63] However, within a clinical setting a response pattern can be quickly detected identifying evening (or morning) types, which can be important information for differential diagnoses and treatment approaches. The M/E has been translated into multiple languages.

Pediatric Daytime Sleepiness Scale

The 8-item Pediatric Daytime Sleepiness Scale (PDSS) was developed as a self-report measure of sleepiness in adolescents ages 11 to 15 years and was further validated for children ages 5 to 17 years.[64,65] The PDSS has been shown to be valid and reliable, and is useful as a clinical screener for sleepiness, and can be used to monitor treatment outcomes.[64,66] The PDSS has been translated into multiple languages, and a recent study from Brazil identified a clinical cutoff score of 15 to indicate significant sleepiness.[67]

Pediatric Insomnia Severity Index

The Pediatric Insomnia Severity Index (PISI) was developed by a multidisciplinary team of pediatric sleep specialists to assess the diagnostic symptoms of insomnia. The PISI is a parent-report measure for children ages 4 to 10 years and has 6 items that assess sleep-onset latency, difficulties with sleep initiation, nighttime awakenings, daytime sleepiness, and sleep duration.[68] Although there are no cutoff scores for the 2 subscales (sleep-onset and sleep-maintenance), if given before a clinic visit, this measure can be quickly scored to provide information for a clinical conversation, as well as to track treatment progress over time.[68]

Pediatric Sleep Practices Questionnaire

The Pediatric Sleep Practices Questionnaire (PSPQ) is a self-report measure for children and adolescents, ages 8 to 17 years, with a parent proxy version for children 5 to 7 years.[16] The PSPQ was developed to screen for sleep practices (or behaviors) that may promote or inhibit sleep and includes 5 factors: sleep timing, sleep routines and consistency, technology use before bedtime, sleep environment, and parental presence to fall asleep. Although there is no total score or clinical cutoff, this measure is useful for identifying poor sleep health behaviors or sleep environments that may be negatively affecting sleep.

Patient-Reported Outcomes Measurement Information System (PROMIS) Pediatric Sleep Disturbance and Sleep-Related Impairment

The Patient-Reported Outcomes Measurement Information System (PROMIS) item banks were developed and validated as part of a larger initiative to support patient-centered health care.[69] Two item banks were developed to assess pediatric sleep, Sleep Disturbances (SD) and Sleep-Related Impairment (SRI). The PROMIS Pediatric SD item bank includes 15 self-report items that assess sleep disturbance and sleep quality in children ages 8 to 17 years (with a parent-proxy version for children ages 5–7 years), and the PROMIS Pediatric SRI item bank includes 13 items that assess daytime sleepiness and daytime functioning related to sleep.[7,70] There are also validated 4- and 8-item short forms, and the total score from each version can be converted to a standardized T-score (mean 50, standard deviation of 10). In addition to validation in the general population and sleep clinic, the PROMIS Pediatric SD and SRI measures have been validated in populations of children with chronic illnesses and developmental disorders.[7,8,71] Recently, these item banks were also validated in young children ages 1 to 5 years.[72] Because of the overlap in items between the young child, pediatric, and adult versions, the PROMIS SD and SRI measures can be used to assess sleep across the lifespan.

Sleep Disturbance Scale for Children

The Sleep Disturbance Scale for Children (SDSC) was developed as a screening measure for common sleep disturbances in children and adolescents (6–16 years). With 26 items, the measure includes 6 factors—disorders of initiating and maintaining sleep, sleep breathing disorders, disorders of arousal, sleep-wake transitions, disorders of excessive somnolence, and sleep hyperhidrosis—and has a recommended cutoff of 39 and provides corresponding T-scores for the total score and factors.[73] As the measure was developed for typically developing children presenting in a sleep clinic, a more recent confirmatory factor analysis focused on children with a range of neurodevelopmental conditions and identified a 5-factor model (excluding sleep hyperhidrosis and one additional item).[74] The SDSC has been translated into multiple languages, and additional studies have validated the SDSC for infants, toddlers, and preschoolers.[75,76]

CLINICAL APPLICATION OF PATIENT-REPORTED QUESTIONNAIRES TO IDENTIFY SLEEP PROFILES

One concern with the use of questionnaires in a clinical setting is the time it takes to score and interpret these measures. However, this last section reviews case examples of how a combination of patient-reported questionnaires can be quickly scanned to identify potential sleep profiles of common presenting sleep problems for patients 8 to 17 years. In our clinic, we use a combination of the PROMIS Pediatric SD and SRI 4-item short forms, 7 items from the PSPQ, the DBAS-10C, and the M/E questionnaire. Together these 31 items typically take children and adolescents 5 to 10 minutes to complete. (Names and ages of patient in the following profiles have been changed).

Frequent Night Wakings and Poor-Quality Sleep

Caroline was a 14-year-old girl who presented with complaints of frequent night wakings and poor-quality sleep. A scan of the PROMIS Pediatric SD and SRI showed significant sleep disturbances ("Almost Always" responses for problems with sleep and trouble sleeping and "Almost Never" for sleeping through the night) and impaired daytime functioning ("Almost Always" sleepy, difficulties with concentrating and getting things done because sleepy, and problems during the day because of poor sleep). However, her PSPQ responses suggested that she "Always" or "Almost Always" had a consistent bedtime, bedtime routine, and wake time, and "Almost Never" used electronics before sleep onset, suggesting this was not simply a matter of sleep hygiene. On the DBAS-10C, she marked "Agree" or "Strongly Agree" on 6 of the 10 items, highlighting beliefs about how her sleep is negatively affecting her daytime functioning. Finally, on the M/E, she selected responses that suggested that she was neither a morning lark nor a night owl, with age-appropriate preferences for bedtimes and wake times and no significant issues in the morning. These data suggest the potential for sleep-maintenance insomnia, other factors that may be interfering with sleep (eg, anxiety), but not poor sleep health behaviors or a delayed circadian sleep-wake rhythm. The detailed clinical interview supported this profile, as Caroline had a history of posttraumatic stress disorder and nightmares, which resulted in frequent nighttime awakenings and subsequent poor daytime functioning.

Difficulty Falling Asleep

Anthony was a 9-year-old boy who presented with difficulty falling asleep. A scan of his questionnaires suggested moderate sleep disturbances ("Sometimes" sleeping through the night, having problems with sleep, trouble sleep but "Almost Always" having difficulty falling asleep), low daytime impairment ("Almost Never" responses for all

PROMIS Pediatric SRI questions), and relatively good sleep health behaviors (consistent bedtime, bedtime routine, and wake time and almost no use of electronics before bedtime). However, it was notable that he selected "Almost Always" needing someone with him to fall asleep, suggesting a sleep-onset association. The scan of his DBAS-10C showed that he agreed with statements about needing to try harder to sleep and worries about how not getting enough sleep might affect his ability to sleep in the future or his daytime functioning. His M/E responses suggested that he was neither a morning lark nor a night owl, selecting age-appropriate preferences for bedtimes and wake times and indicating no significant issues in the morning. Together these responses highlight a profile of sleep-onset insomnia, with some sleep-related anxiety. The detailed clinical history further identified that Anthony had a history of not falling asleep on a couple of occasions until around 4:00 AM and since then had become very anxious about sleep. He would often watch the clock and call out frequently to his parents to let them know he was still awake. However, until directly asked about sleep location (based on the PSPQ response), parents did not report that Anthony was falling asleep on the couch in his parents' room several nights per week or that his parents would often come into his room at bedtime and remain present until he was asleep.

Difficulty Falling Asleep and Difficulty Waking up

Jenna was a 16-year-old girl who presented with difficulties falling asleep and difficulty waking up. Her sleep questionnaires showed a pattern of general few sleep disturbances ("Sometimes" difficulty falling asleep, "Always" sleeping through the night, "Almost Never" problems or trouble with sleeping) and low-to-moderate daytime impairment ("Sometimes" sleepy or having a hard time getting things done, "Never/Almost Never" having a hard time concentrating or problems during the day due to sleep). She reported "Always" having a consistent bedtime routine, "Sometimes" having a consistent bedtime and wake time, "Almost Never" using electronics prior to bedtime, and "Never" needing someone present to fall asleep. Her responses on the DBAS-10C were mostly "Disagree" or "Strongly Disagree," with only "Agree" for 3 items related to how getting insufficient sleep duration affects her during the day. On the M/E questionnaire she consistently selected responses with an evening circadian preference. Together these responses

suggest a profile consistent with a delayed circadian sleep-wake rhythm, with few concerns related to insomnia or poor sleep health. In clinic, she reported significant difficulties falling asleep before 2:00 AM and difficulties waking at 8:30 AM for school but sleeping well on weekends and holidays. At a follow-up visit, when allowed to sleep on her preferred sleep schedule (2:00 AM–11:00 AM) over a school break, she reported no difficulties with falling asleep, waking up, or daytime functioning.

Difficulty Falling Asleep, Difficulty Waking in the Morning, Falling Asleep in Class

Gus was a 15-year-old boy who presented with difficulties falling asleep, difficulties waking in the morning, and reports that he was falling asleep in class. He reported moderate-to-high sleep disturbances ("Almost Always" having problems with or trouble sleeping, "Sometimes" difficulty falling asleep, and "Almost Never" sleeping through the night), very significant daytime impairment ("Always" selected for all PROMIS Pediatric SRI questions), and poor sleep health behaviors ("Never" having a consistent bedtime, bedtime routine, or wake time; "Always" watching videos before falling asleep; and "Sometimes" using an electronic device before falling asleep). He selected "Agree" or "Strongly Agree" on 8 of the 10 DBAS-10C items, with lower ratings only for the 2 items related to needing to nap or stay in bed if unable to sleep at night. His M/E responses suggested some night owl tendencies but bed times, wake times, and time of being alert responses suggesting in general an intermediate type. Together this profile suggests a combination of poor sleep health behaviors and anxiety-related insomnia. In the clinical interview, it was revealed that Gus had significant anxiety following a school shooting, which was impairing his ability to fall asleep or return to sleep following multiple nighttime awakenings. As a result, he would cope with this anxiety at night by playing video games or watching videos until he fell asleep and was unable to maintain a consistent sleep-wake schedule, resulting in the noted daytime impairment.

SUMMARY

Sleep is essential for health and well-being, and all clinicians should routinely screen for sleep health and sleep problems. This chapter provided a number of different considerations for how to screen for sleep within primary care or specialty care practice, including screening questions, clinical interview questions, prospective sleep diaries, and the use of screening questionnaires to identify potential sleep issues. In particular, if filled out ahead of a clinic visit, sleep diaries and sleep questionnaires can provide a wealth of information for clinicians, including targeted questions to assist with differential diagnoses and treatment recommendations.

CLINICS CARE POINTS

- It is important for all clinical providers to ask about sleep problems, with questions directed toward children older than 8 years, as parents may not always be aware of the child's sleep issues.
- When asking about sleep, clinicians should remember that this is not a unidimensional behavior. Instead, questions should focus on the timing, duration, quality, and satisfaction with sleep, as well as behaviors that promote or inhibit sleep.
- When possible, families should complete 1 to 2 weeks of a prospective sleep diary to help clinicians with differential diagnoses and to monitor progress with treatment recommendations.
- Clinicians should select questionnaires that are appropriate for their population and use these measures to help guide diagnoses and treatment planning.

DISCLOSURE

The authors have nothing to disclose.

REFERENCES

1. Meltzer LJ, Williamson AA, Mindell JA. Pediatric sleep health: it matters, and so does how we define it. Sleep Med Rev 2021;57:101425.
2. Sadeh A, Anders TF. Infant sleep problems: origins, assessment, interventions. Infant Ment Health J 1993;14(1):17–34.
3. Newton AT, Honaker SM, Reid GJ. Risk and protective factors and processes for behavioral sleep problems among preschool and early school-aged children: a systematic review. Sleep Med Rev 2020;52:101303.
4. Williamson AA, Meltzer LJ, Fiks AG. A stimulus package to address the pediatric sleep debt crisis in the United States. JAMA Pediatr 2020;174(2):115–6.
5. Meltzer LJ, Crabtree VM. Pediatric sleep problems: a clinician's guide to behavioral interventions. Washington, D.C.: American Psychological Association; 2015.
6. Quach J, Hiscock H, Ukoumunne OC, et al. A brief sleep intervention improves outcomes in the school entry year: a randomized controlled trial. Pediatrics 2011;128(4):692–701.
7. Forrest CB, Meltzer LJ, Marcus CL, et al. Development and validation of the PROMIS pediatric sleep disturbance and sleep-related impairment item banks. Sleep 2018;41(6).
8. Meltzer LJ, Forrest CB, de la Motte A, et al. Clinical validity of the PROMIS pediatric sleep measures across populations of children with chronic illnesses and neurodevelopment disorders. J Pediatr Psychol 2020;45(3):319–27.
9. Mindell JA, Collins M, Leichman ES, et al. Caregiver perceptions of sleep problems and desired areas of change in young children. Sleep Med 2022;92:67–72.
10. Meltzer LJ. Pediatric sleep. In: Youngstrom EA, Prinstein MJ, Mash EJ, et al, editors. Assessment of disorders in childhood and adolescence. 5th edition. New York: Guilford Press; 2020.
11. Stowe RC, Afolabi-Brown O. Pediatric polysomnography-A review of indications, technical aspects, and interpretation. Paediatr Respir Rev 2020;34:9–17.
12. Meltzer LJ. Question 2: when is actigraphy useful for the diagnosis and treatment of sleep problems? Paediatr Respir Rev 2018;28:41–6.
13. Paruthi S, Brooks LJ, D'Ambrosio C, et al. Recommended amount of sleep for pediatric populations: a consensus statement of the American Academy of sleep medicine. J Clin Sleep Med 2016;12(6):785–6.
14. Jenni OG, Carskadon MA. Normal human sleep at different ages: infants to adolescents. In: Opp MR, editor. *SRS basics of sleep guide*. Westchester, IL: Sleep Researcher Society; 2005. p. 11–9.
15. Bronfenbrenner U. The ecology of human development: experiments by nature and design. Cambridge, MA: Harvard University Press; 1979.
16. Meltzer LJ, Forrest CB, de la Motte A, et al. Development and validation of the Pediatric Sleep Practices Questionnaire: a self-report measure for youth ages 8-17 years. Behav Sleep Med 2021;19(1):126–43.
17. Mindell JA, Williamson AA. Benefits of a bedtime routine in young children: sleep, development, and beyond. Sleep Med Rev 2018;40:93–108.
18. Mindell JA, Li AM, Sadeh A, et al. Bedtime routines for young children: a dose-dependent association with sleep outcomes. Sleep 2015;38(5):717–22.
19. Mindell JA, Meltzer LJ, Carskadon MA, et al. Developmental aspects of sleep hygiene: findings from the 2004 national sleep foundation sleep in America poll. Sleep Med 2009;10(7):771–9.
20. Williamson AA, Mindell JA, Hiscock H, et al. Child sleep behaviors and sleep problems from infancy to school-age. Sleep Med 2019;63:5–8.
21. Ahluwalia N, Herrick K. Caffeine intake from food and beverage sources and trends among children

and adolescents in the United States: review of national quantitative studies from 1999 to 2011. Adv Nutr 2015;6(1):102–11.

22. Bruni O, Sette S, Fontanesi L, et al. Technology use and sleep quality in preadolescence and adolescence. J Clin Sleep Med 2015;11(12):1433–41.

23. Mitchell DC, Knight CA, Hockenberry J, et al. Beverage caffeine intakes in the U.S. Food Chem Toxicol 2014;63:136–42.

24. Williamson AA, Milaniak I, Watson B, et al. Early childhood sleep intervention in urban primary care: caregiver and clinician perspectives. J Pediatr Psychol 2020;45(8):933–45.

25. Buysse DJ. Sleep health: can we define it? Does it matter? Sleep 2014;37(1):9–17.

26. Wiggs L, Montgomery P, Stores G. Actigraphic and parent reports of sleep patterns and sleep disorders in children with subtypes of attention-deficit hyperactivity disorder. Sleep 2005;28(11):1437–45.

27. Hvolby A, Jorgensen J, Bilenberg N. Actigraphic and parental reports of sleep difficulties in children with attention-deficit/hyperactivity disorder. Arch Pediatr Adolesc Med 2008;162(4):323–9.

28. Goodlin-Jones BL, Waters S, Anders TF. Objective sleep measurement in typically and atypically developing preschool children with ADHD-like profiles. Child Psychiatr Hum Dev 2009;40(2):257–68.

29. Staton S, Rankin PS, Harding M, et al. Many naps, one nap, none: a systematic review and meta-analysis of napping patterns in children 0-12 years. Sleep Med Rev 2019;50:101247.

30. Short MA, Gradisar M, Lack LC, et al. Estimating adolescent sleep patterns: parent reports versus adolescent self-report surveys, sleep diaries, and actigraphy. Nat Sci Sleep 2013;5:23–6.

31. Combs D, Goodwin JL, Quan SF, et al. Mother knows best? Comparing child report and parent report of sleep parameters with polysomnography. J Clin Sleep Med 2019;15(1):111–7.

32. Mazza S, Bastuji H, Rey AE. Objective and subjective assessments of sleep in children: comparison of actigraphy, sleep diary completed by children and parents' estimation. Front Psychiatry 2020;11: 495.

33. Meltzer LJ, Montgomery-Downs HE, Insana SP, et al. Use of actigraphy for assessment in pediatric sleep research. Sleep Med Rev 2012;16:463–75.

34. Meltzer LJ, Walsh CM, Traylor J, et al. Direct comparison of two new actigraphs and polysomnography in children and adolescents. Sleep 2012;35(1): 159–66.

35. Marcus CL, Brooks LJ, Draper KA, et al. Diagnosis and management of childhood obstructive sleep apnea syndrome. Pediatrics 2012;130(3):576–84.

36. Crowley SJ, Wolfson AR, Tarokh L, et al. An update on adolescent sleep: new evidence informing the perfect storm model. J Adolesc 2018;67:55–65.

37. Buxton OM, Chang AM, Spilsbury JC, et al. Sleep in the modern family: protective family routines for child and adolescent sleep. Sleep Health 2015; 1(1):15–27.

38. Becker SP, Sidol CA, Van Dyk TR, et al. Intraindividual variability of sleep/wake patterns in relation to child and adolescent functioning: a systematic review. Sleep Med Rev 2017;34:94–121.

39. Bei B, Manber R, Allen NB, et al. Too long, too short, or too variable? Sleep intraindividual variability and its associations with perceived sleep quality and mood in adolescents during naturalistically unconstrained sleep. Sleep 2017;40(2).

40. Meltzer LJ, Wainer A, Engstrom E, et al. Seeing the whole elephant: a scoping review of behavioral treatments for pediatric insomnia. Sleep Med Rev 2020;56:101410.

41. Akacem LD, Simpkin CT, Carskadon MA, et al. The timing of the circadian clock and sleep differ between napping and non-napping toddlers. PLoS One 2015;10(4):e0125181.

42. Carney CE, Buysse DJ, Ancoli-Israel S, et al. The consensus sleep diary: standardizing prospective sleep self-monitoring. Sleep 2012;35(2):287–302.

43. Sen T, Spruyt K. Pediatric sleep tools: an updated literature review. Front Psychiatry 2020;11:317.

44. Owens JA, Dalzell V. Use of the 'BEARS' sleep screening tool in a pediatric residents' continuity clinic: a pilot study. Sleep Med 2005;6:63–9.

45. Sadeh A. A brief screening questionnaire for infant sleep problems: validation and findings for an Internet sample. Pediatrics 2004;113(6):e570–7.

46. Mindell JA, Gould RA, Tikotzy L, et al. Norm-referenced scoring system for the brief infant sleep questionnaire - revised (BISQ-R). Sleep Med 2019;63: 106–14.

47. Mindell JA, Du Mond CE, Sadeh A, et al. Efficacy of an internet-based intervention for infant and toddler sleep disturbances. Sleep 2011;34(4):451–8.

48. Mindell JA, Du Mond CE, Sadeh A, et al. Long-term efficacy of an internet-based intervention for infant and toddler sleep disturbances: one year follow-up. J Clin Sleep Med 2011;7(5):507–11.

49. Owens JA, Spirito A, McGuinn M. The Children's Sleep Habits Questionnaire (CSHQ): psychometric properties of a survey instrument for school-aged children. Sleep 2000;23(8):1043–51.

50. Goodlin-Jones BL, Sitnick SL, Tang K, et al. The Children's Sleep Habits Questionnaire in toddlers and preschool children. J Dev Behav Pediatr 2008; 29(2):82–8.

51. Sneddon P, Peacock GG, Crowley SL. Assessment of sleep problems in preschool aged children: an adaptation of the children's sleep habits questionnaire. Behav Sleep Med 2013;11(4):283–96.

52. Bonuck KA, Goodlin-Jones BL, Schechter C, et al. Modified Children's sleep habits questionnaire for

behavioral sleep problems: a validation study. Sleep Health 2017;3(3):136–41.

53. Morin CM, Vallieres A, Ivers H. Dysfunctional beliefs and attitudes about sleep (DBAS): validation of a brief version (DBAS-16). Sleep 2007;30(11): 1547–54.

54. Gregory AM, Cox J, Crawford MR, et al. Dysfunctional beliefs and attitudes about sleep in children. J Sleep Res 2009;18(4):422–6.

55. Blunden S, Gregory AM, Crawford MR. Development of a short version of the dysfunctional beliefs about sleep questionnaire for use with children (DBAS-C10). J Sleep Disord Treat Care 2013;2(3). Available at: https://www.scitechnol.com/development-short-version-dysfunctional-beliefs-about-sleep-questionnaire-use-with-children-dbasc-rXIc.php?article_id=1391.

56. Johns MW. A new method for measuring daytime sleepiness: the Epworth sleepiness scale. Sleep 1991;14(6):540–5.

57. Johns MW. Reliability and factor analysis of the Epworth sleepiness scale. Sleep 1992;15(4):376–81.

58. Melendres MCS, Lutz JM, Rubin ED, et al. Daytime sleepiness and hyperactivity in children with suspected sleep-disordered breathing. Pediatrics 2004;114(3):768–75.

59. Garetz SL, Mitchell RB, Parker PD, et al. Quality of life and obstructive sleep apnea symptoms after pediatric adenotonsillectomy. Pediatrics 2015;135(2): e477–86.

60. Janssen KC, Phillipson S, O'Connor J, et al. Validation of the Epworth sleepiness scale for children and adolescents using rasch analysis. Sleep Med 2017;33:30–5.

61. Carskadon MA, Acebo C. Relationship of a morningess/eveningness scale to sleep patterns in children. Sleep Res 1992;21:367.

62. Carskadon MA, Vieira C, Acebo C. Association between puberty and delayed phase preference. Sleep 1993;16(3):258–62.

63. Diaz-Morales JF, de Leon MC, Sorroche MG. Validity of the morningness-eveningness scale for children among Spanish adolescents. Chronobiol Int 2007; 24(3):435–47.

64. Drake C, Nickel C, Burduvali E, et al. The pediatric daytime sleepiness scale (PDSS): sleep habits and school outcomes in middle-school children. Sleep 2003;26(4):455–8.

65. Meyer C, Ferrari GJJ, Barbosa DG, et al. Analysis of daytime sleepiniess in adolescents by the pediatric daytime sleepiness scale: a systematic review. Rev Paul Pediatr 2017;35(3):351–60.

66. Perez-Chada D, Perez-Lloret S, Videla AJ, et al. Sleep disordered breathing and daytime sleepiness are associated with poor academic performance in teenagers. A study using the Pediatric Daytime Sleepiness Scale (PDSS). Sleep 2007;30(12): 1698–703.

67. Meyer C, Barbosa DG, Junior GJF, et al. Proposal of cutoff points for pediatric daytime sleepiness scale to identify excessive daytime sleepiness. Chronobiol Int 2018;35(3):303–11.

68. Byars KC, Simon SL, Peugh J, et al. Validation of a brief insomnia severity measure in youth clinically referred for sleep evaluation. J Pediatr Psychol 2017;42(4):466–75.

69. Cella D, Yount S, Rothrock N, et al. The Patient-Reported Outcomes Measurement Information System (PROMIS): progress of an NIH Roadmap cooperative group during its first two years. Med Care 2007;45(5 Suppl 1):S3–11.

70. Bevans KB, Meltzer LJ, De La Motte A, et al. Qualitative development and content validation of the PROMIS pediatric sleep health items. Behav Sleep Med 2019;17(5):657–71.

71. Daniel LC, Gross JY, Meltzer LJ, et al. Clinical validity of the PROMIS pediatric sleep short forms in children receiving treatment for cancer. Pediatr Blood Cancer 2020;67(9):e28535.

72. Lai JS, Blackwell CK, Tucker CA, et al. Measuring PROMIS(R) physical activity and sleep problems in early childhood. J Pediatr Psychol 2022;47(5): 534–46.

73. Bruni O, Ottaviano S, Guidetti V, et al. The Sleep Disturbance Scale for Children (SDSC) Construction and validation of an instrument to evaluate sleep disturbances in childhood and adolescence. J Sleep Res 1996;5(4):251–61.

74. Marriner AM, Pestell C, Bayliss DM, et al. Confirmatory factor analysis of the Sleep Disturbance Scale for Children (SDSC) in a clinical sample of children and adolescents. J Sleep Res 2017;26(5):587–94.

75. Romeo DM, Bruni O, Brogna C, et al. Application of the sleep disturbance scale for children (SDSC) in preschool age. Eur J Paediatr Neurol 2013;17(4): 374–82.

76. Romeo DM, Cordaro G, Macchione E, et al. Application of the sleep disturbance scale for children (SDSC) in infants and toddlers (6-36 months). Sleep Med 2021;81:62–8.

Control of Breathing and Central Hypoventilation Syndromes

Julie M. Baughn, MD*, Christine A. Matarese, DO

KEYWORDS

- Pediatric • Hypoventilation • Control of breathing • Congenital central hypoventilation syndrome
- Rapid-onset obesity • Hypothalamic dysfunction • Autonomic dysregulation

KEY POINTS

- Control of breathing varies with age and sleep state.
- Central hypoventilation is a feature of several, rare childhood disorders.
- Hypoventilation and other breathing disturbances are features of other disorders presenting in childhood.
- Disorders or structural abnormalities affecting the brainstem may affect control of breathing.

INTRODUCTION

This article provides an overview of control of breathing including relevant anatomy, impact of sleep stage, and a special discussion of control of breathing in infancy. The clinical evaluation of hypoventilation by polysomnography (PSG) is reviewed. There is also a detailed overview of disorders of central hypoventilation including congenital central hypoventilation syndrome (CCHS) and rapid-onset obesity, hypoventilation, hypothalamic dysfunction, and autonomic dysregulation (ROHHAD). Some additional, more common, disorders that may present in childhood and affect control of breathing are be discussed. The clinical features and abnormalities of ventilation observed with these disorders are highlighted.

BACKGROUND: CONTROL OF BREATHING, VENTILATORY RESPONSES, AND THE EFFECT OF SLEEP

Control of breathing affects how we think about the major forms of sleep-disordered breathing in children. The impact of both behavioral (voluntary) and metabolic (involuntary) control of breathing as well as the influence of respiratory muscles are important components of central sleep apnea, obstructive sleep apnea, and sleep-related hypoventilation. Understanding control of breathing and the impact of the stage of sleep on breathing is important as we discuss, in detail, disorders of central hypoventilation in children. The influence and impact of the arousal response adds to the impact of abnormal breathing events during sleep.

In nonrapid eye movement (NREM) sleep, breathing has a decreased frequency and more regular pattern than during wakefulness; this is under metabolic or involuntary control, and response to carbon dioxide (CO_2) and oxygen is present.[1] In rapid eye movement (REM) sleep there is a behavioral impact on control of breathing that may be associated with dreams.[1] Irregular respiratory efforts and muscle atonia contribute to the high risk of sleep-disordered breathing occurring in the sleep state. Wakefulness also has both metabolic and behavioral components. The ability for individuals to hyperventilate with behavioral control is easier than hypoventilating or breath holding. Disorders with an abnormal metabolic control of breathing (ie, CCHS) primarily affect NREM sleep and wakefulness, with REM sleep

Division of Pulmonary and Critical Care, Mayo Clinic Center for Sleep Medicine, Mayo Clinic, 200 First Street Southwest, Rochester, MN 55905, USA
* Corresponding author.
E-mail address: Baughn.Julie@mayo.edu

Sleep Med Clin 18 (2023) 161–171
https://doi.org/10.1016/j.jsmc.2023.01.002
1556-407X/23/© 2023 Elsevier Inc. All rights reserved.

sleep.theclinics.com

being relatively preserved. In CCHS, there is a mutation in the PHOX2B gene. The transcription factor that is normally a product of this gene plays a role in the autonomic nervous system, and without it there is a loss of control of automatic breathing.[2]

In response to increased partial pressure of CO2, ventilation will increase via an increased tidal volume followed by an increase in respiratory rate.[3] In response to a decreased partial pressure of oxygen, ventilation will increase but this increase is reduced over time.[3] During REM sleep there is a further reduction in ventilatory muscle tone and an increase in CO2 as well as more respiratory variability due to relatively more input from the motor cortex with relatively less input from the brainstem centers.[3] During sleep, periodic breathing may occur if there is a small difference between the eupneic and apneic thresholds, which commonly occurs in infants.[3]

Anatomy Relevant to the Control of Breathing

Brainstem

The brainstem is an important area involved in the control of breathing. Brainstem compression (for example, from a Chiari malformation, achondroplasia, or trauma) or disorders affecting the brainstem (tumors, metabolic disorders) can affect breathing by disruption of the critical areas involved in the generation of respiration and the ventilatory responses to hypoxia and hypercapnia. The ventrolateral medulla is an important brainstem area involved in regulating respiration and ventilatory responses to changes in CO2 via central chemoreceptors as well as modulation of information from peripheral chemoreceptors and laryngeal afferents.[4] The medullary raphe nucleus (caudal medulla) also is involved in the respiratory response to CO2.[4] The ventral medullary respiratory group is responsible for pacemaker activity and generates the respiratory rhythm.[5] The nucleus tractus solitarius, part of the dorsal medullary respiratory group, integrates central afferents from peripheral chemoreceptors and baroreceptors.[5] The retrotrapezoid nucleus, in the rostral ventral medulla, connects these groups and is the primary respiratory chemoreceptor area.[5] Neurons in this area are sensitive to changes in oxygen and CO2 and receive input from the carotid bodies, hypothalamus, and central pattern generator.[3] The pontine respiratory group influences the preinspiratory and expiratory phases of breathing.[5] These areas are important in the metabolic control of breathing. Disorders affecting the brainstem (ie, Chiari malformation) result in abnormal breathing during NREM sleep, as breathing in this sleep stage is under metabolic control.

Hypothalamus

The hypothalamus is another area involved in the control of breathing. It is an area of gray matter located below the thalamus that is better known for its role in the autonomic nervous system and maintaining homeostasis but it is also involved in sleep and respiration. There are several regions of the hypothalamus that are involved in respiratory control including the paraventricular nucleus, perifornical area, and dorsomedial, lateral, and posterior regions.[6] Disorders such as ROHHAD illustrate the role of the hypothalamus in both the autonomic nervous system and control of breathing. The paraventricular nucleus contains neurons that communicate with other areas involved in the control of breathing, maintains homeostasis, and drives baseline respiration.[6] The paraventricular nucleus mediates the respiratory response to hypoxia; it receives afferents from the nucleus tractus solitarius that receives input from the carotid bodies in response to hypoxia.[6] The perifornical area is involved in regulation of basal respiration and increases respiration in response to alerting stimuli or stressors.[6] The dorsomedial hypothalamus is known as the center for defense response and increases respiration in response to stressors.[6] The lateral hypothalamus is involved in the regulation of breathing and in response to changes in CO2.[6] The posterior hypothalamus is involved in maintaining baseline respiration, has projections to several brain areas involved in respiratory control, and facilitates response to hypoxia.[6]

Arousal response

In addition to brainstem and hypothalamic inputs on control of breathing, the arousal response affects breathing events and is affected by sleep state. This arousal response is important in obstructive sleep apnea in children.[7,8] In obstructive sleep apnea (OSA) the arousal response to an event and/or associated gas exchange abnormality affects the duration of the event and the degree of desaturation. There is a spectrum of obstructive sleep apnea from upper airway resistance syndrome to frequent and cyclic obstruction that is likely affected by control of breathing. In children control of breathing is relatively preserved, and events can occur without significant sleep disruption.

Neonatal/infant control of breathing

Disorders affecting the control of breathing, such as the central hypoventilation disorder CCHS, can present as early as the neonatal period. A discussion of control of breathing during the neonatal period and infancy is important because during this stage of rapid development there are corresponding rapid changes that occur in breathing; this makes the identification of sleep-disordered breathing challenging in this age group, as what is considered normal at one age may not be considered normal a few weeks later.

The central nervous system and respiratory mechanics are not fully developed at birth and undergo continued development and organization over time. This immaturity or incomplete development affects respiratory effort and ventilatory responses.

In the fetus, the lungs are fluid-filled, and the diaphragm is the primary muscle of breathing.[9] A feedback system exists even at this early stage of development, and the central chemoreceptors adjust ventilatory responses based on CO_2 levels and pH.[9] Hypoxia depresses respiratory movements, and cycles of respiratory activity are correlated with the sleep/wake cycle.[9]

Following delivery, the infant transitions from a fluid-filled state to breathing air. The diaphragm generates a negative pressure to initiate respiration, fluid is cleared from the lungs, and the functional residual capacity of the lungs increases over the first few days of life.[9] The central chemoreceptors respond to CO_2 similarly as in adults (minute ventilation increases with increased CO_2), and the peripheral chemoreceptors adjust to an increase in the partial pressure of oxygen in the first few days of life.[9]

In the neonate, the respiratory centers are immature, the airway is relatively narrow and susceptible to collapse, the muscles in the chest wall are weak, and there is a mechanical disadvantage due to the shape and increased compliance of the chest wall.[9] The functional residual capacity of the lungs is low, and ventilation is maintained by increasing respiratory rate.[9] Reflex induced apnea occurs in response to stimulation of the laryngeal mucosa, mediated through superior laryngeal nerve afferents, and this response is exaggerated in preterm infants.[4] Hypoxia decreases the response to CO_2 levels; there is an initial increase in ventilation followed by a decrease, which decreases metabolism and allows for better tolerance of hypoxia.[9] This decrease in metabolism in response to hypoxia also decreases CO_2 levels and if less than the apneic threshold, will cause apnea.[10] The initial increase in ventilation is due to stimulation of the peripheral chemoreceptors, and the subsequent decrease in ventilation is caused by a decrease in respiratory rate with the tidal volume remaining steady.[4]

In premature infants, control of breathing is immature, and hypotonia, periodic breathing, irregular breathing, and central apnea are common.[9] Apnea causes a decrease in the partial pressure of oxygen, the extent of which is related to the duration of the apnea and the baseline partial pressure of oxygen.[4] In response to hypoxia there is an initial increase in ventilation followed by a decrease.[4] Neurotransmitters including adenosine are involved in hypoxia-induced respiratory depression, and treatment with methylxanthines (theophylline and caffeine), which block adenosine, is used in the management of apnea of prematurity.[4] Methylxanthines improve CO_2 sensitivity, decrease periodic breathing, increase minute ventilation, and decrease hypoxic respiratory depression.[4] Control of breathing improves as the respiratory centers mature but apnea of prematurity can still be seen at 44 weeks.[11] Preterm infants are also predisposed to central apnea/periodic breathing because their eupneic and apneic thresholds (level of CO_2 less than which breathing ceases) are close together.[11] Small variations in respiration may result in the level of CO_2 becoming less than the apneic threshold, resulting in apnea or periodic breathing. Irregular baseline breathing, which is common in neonates, also affects the partial pressure of oxygen, and small changes in O_2 can result in large changes in ventilation due to the relatively increased response of the peripheral chemoreceptors at this age.[10]

Clinical Evaluation of Hypoventilation in Children

Sleep-related hypoventilation

When sleep-related hypoventilation is observed in children, this diagnosis should prompt consideration of one of the disorders of central hypoventilation, particularly in the absence of another cause. A thorough evaluation of the cardiac, pulmonary, and neurologic systems is recommended, which may include imaging of the brain and brainstem, echocardiogram, pulmonary function test, and an evaluation for neuromuscular disease. Elevated CO_2 can be seen in OSA. Children with obesity can have mildly elevated CO_2 levels, which may be associated with comorbid OSA (obstructive hypoventilation). It should be noted that obesity hypoventilation syndrome is not well described in the literature in children. The presence of significantly increased CO_2, especially associated with significant hypoxemia, should prompt further evaluation for a central hypoventilation syndrome.

The AASM Scoring manual recommends measuring CO_2 with either transcutaneous, end-tidal, or arterial blood gas in association with the evaluation of children by polysomnography and defines sleep-related hypoventilation as at least a quarter of the total sleep time having a CO_2 greater than 50 mm Hg by one of these measurements.[12] The use and familiarity with each of these measures of CO_2 is important for the pediatric sleep medicine provider to accurately identify and diagnose children with hypoventilation. Each of these measures has features that can affect its accuracy. There is frequent need for recalibration of transcutaneous CO_2, and it can lag behind actual arterial CO_2. There is a tendency for it to trend upward over time, especially without recalibration due to warming of the skin and local CO_2 production. End-tidal CO_2 can also be inaccurate and is difficult to interpret in the setting of supplemental oxygen use or positive airway pressure. The measurement of arterial CO_2 in children can be difficult. Often capillary blood gases are obtained in children because when done correctly they approximate arterial CO_2. Whether the child is awake or asleep during the attainment of this value, as well as if they are crying (leading to hyperventilation and a lower CO_2 than expected) affect the results. Clinical correlation and interpretation by the provider are necessary when these methods of CO_2 monitoring are used.[12]

Oximetry during PSG can also suggest hypoventilation. Baseline saturations less than 95 suggest hypoventilation in the setting of normal pulmonary and cardiac systems. This feature is seen in children with neuromuscular disease or hypotonia. Hypopneas observed that are not associated with obstructive features can also suggest hypoventilation, particularly in REM sleep. These features on PSG are commonly seen when evaluating children with neuromuscular weakness or hypotonia. Most forms of hypoventilation or sleep-disordered breathing will be worse in REM sleep. OSA is often predominant or worse in REM sleep. Sleep-related hypoventilation related to neuromuscular disease or other forms of restrictive lung disease typically occurs first in REM sleep before involving non-REM sleep and wakefulness.

The presence of central sleep apnea in non-REM sleep suggests abnormal control of breathing, and further evaluation is needed. It is important to note, however, that normal central apneas and central pauses are quite common in typical children and are not a cause for concern. Brief (typically <10 seconds) central apneas are normal in children in REM sleep. These events can meet scoring criteria because they may be associated with an oxygen fluctuation of 3%. In addition, non-REM postsigh/postarousal central apneas also occur and may meet scoring criteria yet still be normal. Prolonged and/or repetitive central apneas in NREM sleep are abnormal and require further investigation.

There are clinical features that should raise suspicion for hypoventilation and in some cases abnormal control of breathing, independent of polysomnography; these include recurrent respiratory illnesses that require hospitalization and/or a history of respiratory failure associated with a viral illness or anesthesia. This clinical history may be the presenting sign of a central hypoventilation syndrome, such as later-onset CCHS (LO-CCHS) or ROHHAD.[2]

Disorders of central hypoventilation
There is a significant clinical overlap between the most common disorders of central hypoventilation and disorders with hypothalamic dysfunction. The following sections review key clinical features of these disorders. Please refer to **Fig. 1** (clinical overlap and differences seen in ROHHAD, LO-CCHS, and Prader-Willi Syndrome [PWS]) and **Table 1** (clinical features of CCHS, LO-CCHS, and ROHHAD).

Congenital central hypoventilation syndrome
The International Classification of Sleep Disorders, 3rd Edition (ICSD-3) classifies CCHS by the following 2 criteria:[13]

- The presence of sleep-related hypoventilation
- A mutation in the PHOX2B gene

Genetics of congenital central hypoventilation syndrome
CCHS is due to a mutation in the PHOX2B gene. This gene is highly conserved across species and affects the autonomic nervous system. The normal pattern is a 20-alanine repeat sequence. Individuals with CCHS will have an autosomal dominant polyalanine repeat expansion mutation (PARM). A small percentage of individuals with CCHS will have a non-PARM mutation (missense, nonsense, or frameshift mutation).[14,15] All parents of children with CCHS should be tested, as there can be parental mosaicism. Lower polyalanine repeat mutations may require an additional environmental stimulus to reveal evidence of hypoventilation, which can include sedation, anesthesia, or respiratory illness.[14,16] These individuals are often described as those with LO-CCHS.

Key clinical features of congenital central hypoventilation syndrome
Neonatal-onset CCHS (symptoms occurring in the first 30 days of life) is the more common and "classic" presentation of CCHS and manifests as hypoventilation with sleep only or with sleep and wakefulness. Shallow, monotonous respiratory rates are noted with significantly elevated CO_2 as well as significant hypoxemia. Later-onset

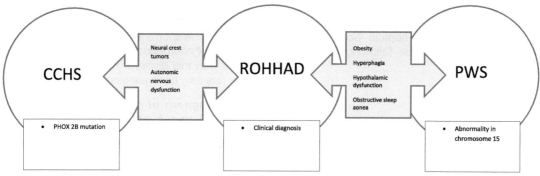

Fig. 1. Intrinsic and overlapping features of disorders with central hypoventilation.

CCHS occurs after the first 30 days of life. It is differentiated from ROHHAD due to the presence of a mutation in the PHOX2B gene and may require an environmental stimulus to reveal the disordered control of breathing.

In a recent review of 72 patients with CCHS it was observed that almost one-third had evidence of Hirschsprung disease. Most of them were associated with a 20/27 PARM mutation but this was not an exclusive mutation that was found with Hirschsprung disease.[17] In addition, it has been identified that individuals with CCHS can have symptomatic and asymptomatic cardiac pauses requiring pacemaker placement due to potential life-threatening arrhythmias.[18]

Table 1
Presenting and key clinical features of CCHS, LO-CCHS, and ROHHAD

Features	CCHS	LO-CCHS	ROHHAD
Presenting features	Cyanosis, hypoventilation during sleep, shallow breathing, asymptomatic in the face of hypoxia, hypercapnia	May present in childhood or beyond, with respiratory depression following sedation or illness, asymptomatic in the face of hypoxia, hypercapnia	Hypoventilation during sleep, asymptomatic in the face of hypoxia, hypercapnia
PSG	Hypoventilation during sleep (worse in NREM), shallow respirations	Hypoventilation during sleep, central sleep apnea	Hypoventilation during sleep, OSA
Cardiac	Arrhythmias, sinus pauses, prolonged QTc, asystole, orthostatic hypotension	Cor pulmonale	Can cause cardiorespiratory arrest
Autonomic nervous system/neural crest	Associated with Hirschsprung disease and neural crest tumors	Associated with Hirschsprung disease and neural crest tumors	Autonomic dysfunction (temperature dysregulation, decreased pain sensation, diarrhea/constipation) Associated with neural crest tumors
Hypothalamic dysfunction	Not prominent	Not prominent	Prominent (hyperphagia, obesity, delayed or precocious puberty, sodium imbalance)

Because of the multisystem impact of this disease, periodic surveillance has been recommended by the American Thoracic Society[16] and includes evaluation of the following at regular intervals.

- PSG
- Echocardiogram
- Routine laboratory evaluation
- Prolonged electrocardiogram monitoring
- Neurocognitive testing
- Screening for neural crest tumors

Many children need respiratory support during both sleep and wakefulness, and this depends on the mutation or degree of polyalanine repeats present. Some may need support only during sleep. Support may include tracheostomy and ventilation, diaphragmatic pacing, and noninvasive positive airway pressure ventilation.

Rapid-Onset Obesity, Hypothalamic Dysfunction, Hypoventilation, and Autonomic Dysregulation

The ICSD-3 classifies ROHHAD by the following criteria[13]:

- Presence of sleep-related hypoventilation
- Presentation after the first few years of life
- At least 2 of the following clinical features:
  ○ Obesity
  ○ Hypothalamic endocrine dysfunction
  ○ Emotional and behavioral disturbances
  ○ Neural crest tumor
- Absence of a PHOX2B mutation
- The absence of another explanation for the findings

ROHHAD was first described as a syndrome by Ize-Ludlow and colleagues in 2007,[19] providing nomenclature and a description of a distinct clinical phenotype to patients with both hypothalamic dysfunction and late-onset hypoventilation that had been described in the literature for decades.[20] Its relative recent description and definition as well as the identification of the disease defining mutation of CCHS allowed individuals with ROHHAD to be more readily differentiated from those with LO-CCHS. The relative rarity of this diagnosis and its description in the literature, as well as the clinical nature of the diagnosis make the diagnosis of ROHHAD quite challenging. Its clinical features overlap with aspects of other central hypoventilation disorders including LO-CCHS and PWS. The PSG findings of this disorder are not described in detail in the literature. The presence of hypoventilation can occur after the identification of OSA or emerge after OSA is effectively treated. Central

apnea occurs in some individuals. Other individuals present with acute respiratory failure triggered by a viral illness or anesthesia.[13] Because of the presence of neuroendocrine tumors in some individuals with this disorder ROHHAD nerural crest tumor has also been suggested.[21]

Clinical diagnosis of rapid-onset obesity, hypoventilation, hypothalamic dysfunction, and autonomic dysregulation

Clinical characteristics of ROHHAD include rapid weight gain, hypothalamic and autonomic dysfunction, and central hypoventilation. Presentation is typically in early childhood with hyperphagia and rapid weight gain,[22] following a period of normal development. Various endocrine manifestations of hypothalamic dysfunction present months to years following the rapid onset of obesity.[22] Autonomic dysfunction can manifest as temperature dysregulation, gastrointestinal dysmotility, ophthalmologic abnormalities, and altered pain sensation.[22] Tumors of neural crest origin may develop. Sleep-disordered breathing may occur and can include OSA, central sleep apnea, and hypoventilation. Hypoventilation can be life-threatening, as it can cause cardiorespiratory arrest.[22] An abnormal response to exercise has also been identified and is important to note, as this disorder also affects control of breathing during wakefulness. Prolonged breath holding, for example, during underwater swimming (given the abnormal ventilatory response to hypercapnia) can be dangerous.[19]

Obesity and hypoventilation are present in all individuals with ROHHAD but many of the other clinical features including autonomic dysfunction can have variable presentations.[23] Because this is a rare disorder with overlapping features with other disorders, diagnosis can be a challenge. Evaluation and testing for known mutations in other disorders (ie, PHOX2B) is necessary to rule out other causes. The development of consensus guidelines for the evaluation and treatment of ROHHAD would be of benefit to patients and clinicians.

Disorders Affecting Control of Breathing

Prader-Willi syndrome

PWS is a rare, genetic disorder that, in most cases, is due to a deletion in the paternally derived copy of chromosome 15q11-q13. Clinical features in infants include hypotonia and feeding difficulties. Clinical features in children include hypothalamic dysfunction characterized by hyperphagia, obesity, hypogonadism, growth hormone deficiency/short stature, and dysautonomia as well as behavioral and learning difficulties. Infants with PWS are prone to central sleep apnea.[24]

Sleep-disordered breathing is common in children with PWS and may include the following, which can evolve over time:

- Central sleep apnea
- Obstructive sleep apnea
- Hypoventilation

Ventilatory responses are altered in patients with PWS. The response to decreased O2 (hypoxic ventilatory response) is mediated by peripheral chemoreceptors located in the carotid bodies that communicate with respiratory control centers to affect respiratory rate and tidal volume.[25] The response to elevated blood CO2 levels (hypercapnic ventilatory response) is mediated by the peripheral chemoreceptors as well as central chemoreceptors located in the ventral medulla. These ventilatory responses are blunted in PWS.[25] Hypothalamic dysfunction is a feature of PWS, and hypothalamic nuclei are involved in the control of respiration and in coordinating the response to hypoxemia and hypercapnia.[6] Children with PWS are frequently treated with growth hormone (GH), and GH may modulate the sensitivity of peripheral chemoreceptors to CO2 or affect the communication to central respiratory control centers.[25] A case series of 16 children with PWS published in 2013 by Katz-Salamon and colleagues noted GH treatment increased arterial oxygenation during sleep but did not alter ventilatory chemoreceptor-mediated responsiveness to changes in oxygen or CO2.[26] Treatment with GH may accelerate the growth of tonsillar and adenoid tissue, increasing the risk for obstructive sleep apnea. Because of the variable impact of GH on sleep-disordered breathing in PWS, a PSG before the initiation of GH and again approximately 6 weeks after treatment is initiated is recommended.[27]

Familial dysautonomia

Familial dysautonomia (also known as Riley-Day syndrome) is a rare, autosomal recessive disorder caused by a mutation in the IKBKAP gene that affects the autonomic nervous system. Symptoms include hypotonia, decreased sensitivity to pain and temperature, temperature and blood pressure instability, and lack of tears. Respiratory complications, abnormal ventilatory control/decreased response to hypoxemia, and hypoventilation during sleep are common.[2] In the setting of hypoxia, ventilation in patients with familial dysautonomia initially increases and then decreases.[28] Denervation affecting chemoreceptors and baroreceptors in familial dysautonomia has not been demonstrated but has been speculated.[28] Breath holding, which can be severe and result in cyanosis,

syncope, and decerebrate posturing, is also common in children with familial dysautonomia and may be secondary to insensitivity to hypoxia and hypercapnia.[28]

Leigh syndrome

Leigh syndrome is a rare metabolic disorder that is also known as subacute necrotizing encephalomyelopathy. It can be caused by various gene mutations, most commonly affecting the mitochondrial respiratory chain complex or the pyruvate dehydrogenase complex. Clinical presentation is typically in infancy and early childhood and involves, after a period of normal development, developmental regression, hypotonia, vomiting, dystonia, seizures, lactic acidosis, eye movement abnormalities, and then progressive neurologic decline. The brainstem, basal ganglia, cerebellum, and cerebral cortex are usually affected. Sleep-wake disturbances, apnea, and alveolar hypoventilation may develop, and the hypoventilation may precede other symptoms.[2]

Disorders Affecting the Brainstem

Chiari malformation type 1

Chiari malformation type 1 is the most common type of the Chiari malformations, is usually congenital, and is characterized by downward herniation of the cerebellar tonsils below the plane of the foramen magnum (basion-opisthion line). The posterior fossa is typically small, and this may cause compression of the cerebellum. This rostral displacement of the hindbrain can cause compression of the cerebellum and medulla against the edges of the foramen magnum. Children may be asymptomatic or present with occipital headaches (typically exacerbated by Valsalva or exertion), diplopia, nystagmus, retroorbital pain, dysphagia, and dysarthria. A syrinx (syringomyelia/collection of cerebrospinal fluid [CSF] within the spinal cord) is a common associated condition, and symptoms may include paresthesias and sensory abnormalities over the shoulders, arms, upper trunk, and hand weakness. Sleep-disordered breathing can also occur in association with Chiari malformations and may include central sleep apnea, OSA, and hypoventilation. Several factors may be involved in the development of sleep-disordered breathing including brainstem compression affecting the pontomedullary respiratory network leading to central apneas and traction/compression of the lower cranial nerves leading to hypotonia of the pharyngeal muscles. A prospective study investigating the prevalence of sleep-disordered breathing in 90 (adult) patients with Chiari malformation type 1 was published in 2017 by Ferré and colleagues.[29] They found a high prevalence of sleep-related breathing disorders (50%), predominantly obstructive hypopneas, during REM supine sleep. Six patients had a central apnea index of 5 or more and 3 had hypoventilation.[29] The exact cause of central hypoventilation in Chiari malformations is unknown but support for the concept that brainstem compression can damage the central brainstem pathways controlling respiration and cause nocturnal hypoventilation is found in a case report published in 2005 by Bhangoo and colleagues.[30] Two children developed nocturnal hypoventilation in the setting of acute deterioration of hindbrain-hernia (AKA Chiari malformation type 1)-related syringomyelia despite successful decompression and shunt placement.[30]

Chiari malformation type 2

Chiari malformation type 2 is characterized by displacement of the medulla, fourth ventricle, and cerebellum through the foramen magnum. It is commonly associated with myelomeningocele (an open spinal column), which is evident at birth, and hydrocephalus (due to obstruction of the flow of CSF). Symptoms and sleep-disordered breathing include those seen with type 1 as well as symptoms of hydrocephalus (somnolence, balance problems and incoordination, vomiting, macrocephaly). Infants may present with apnea, bradycardia, and vocal cord dysfunction. Given the medulla's importance in control of breathing, and the involvement of this region in a Chiari malformation type 2, the respiratory centers may be impaired from traction, trauma, or damage related to hydrocephalus.[2] In the study mentioned earlier by Ferré and colleagues, hydrocephalus was associated with the presence and severity of sleep-related breathing disorders.[29]

Achondroplasia

Achondroplasia, although rare, is the most common type of short-limbed dwarfism. It is an autosomal dominant skeletal dysplasia caused by a mutation in the fibroblast growth factor receptor 3 gene.

Clinical features include the following:

- Shortened limb bones
- Short stature
- Hypotonia
- Motor delay
- Macrocephaly
- Midface hypoplasia

Sleep-disordered breathing is common in children with achondroplasia and includes the following:

- Central sleep apnea
- Obstructive sleep apnea
- Hypoventilation

Mogayzel and colleagues published a study in 1998 evaluating sleep-disordered breathing in 88 children younger than 14 years with achondroplasia and found primarily hypoxemia as opposed to central speel apnea or OSA[31]; this may be reflective of restrictive lung disease given their thoracic/rib bony abnormalities. It is also possible that these thoracic abnormalities predispose to hypoventilation. Several children had normal oxygenation and ventilation while awake but hypoxemia and hypercapnia during sleep.[31] Disproportion between the size of the skull and the skull base can increase the risk of brain stem (medullary) compression and resultant central hypoventilation[2] or central sleep apnea.[31] A review of 85 children with achondroplasia was published in 1983 by Stokes and colleagues and noted OSA, hypoxemia, and an autopsy finding of compression of the medulla at the level of the foramen magnum.[32] There may be an abnormal arousal response in these individuals that contributes to a risk of sudden death.[33] It is recommended that individuals with achondroplasia have a PSG in the neonatal period and subsequently based on symptoms.[34]

Acquired causes of central hypoventilation

There are other entities that can cause central hypoventilation during sleep, likely via alteration of CO_2 receptor sensitivity,[35] including space occupying lesions of the brain (tumor or demyelinating disease), ischemia, vascular malformations, trauma, and infection. Children with brain tumors such as medulloblastoma, astrocytoma, and ependymoma and those who have received radiation to the brain are at risk for disorders of respiratory control, including hypoventilation.[2]

Disorders Associated with Apnea and Hyperpnea

Joubert syndrome

Joubert syndrome is a rare genetic disorder characterized by hypoplasia of the cerebellar vermis. It is autosomal recessive and can be caused by mutations in several genes. Children typically present with developmental delay, hypotonia, and ataxia and may have dysmorphic features. Breathing disturbances may occur in some children with Joubert syndrome, particularly during the neonatal period and may include episodes of apnea alternating with tachypnea. A study by Kamdar and colleagues published in 2011 investigated self-reported sleep and breathing disturbances in 20

Table 2
Sleep and breathing abnormalities in disorders affecting ventilation

Disorder	Sleep Findings	Breathing Abnormalities
CCHS	Hypoventilation	Lack of compensatory mechanisms for hypoxia/hypercapnia
ROHHAD	Hypoventilation	Lack of compensatory mechanisms for hypoxia/hypercapnia
Prader-Willi Syndrome	OSA, CSA, hypoventilation	Blunted ventilatory responses to hypoxia and hypercapnia
Achondroplasia	OSA, CSA, hypoventilation	Restrictive lung disease
Chiari malformation type 1	OSA, CSA, hypoventilation	Not prominent
Chiari Malformation Type 2	OSA, CSA, hypoventilation	Not prominent
Leigh syndrome	Hypoventilation apnea	Progressive decline
Familial dysautonomia	Hypoventilation	Blunted ventilatory responses to hypoxia and hypercapnia
Joubert syndrome	Not prominent	Episodes of apnea alternating with tachypnea
Rett syndrome	Not prominent	Prominent feature of the syndrome Episodes of apnea, irregular breathing, and hyperventilation (more prominent during wake than sleep)

patients with Joubert syndrome.[36] Episodic tachypnea was reported in 35%, apnea in 20%, both apnea and tachypnea in 15%, snoring in 50%, and 43% had scores on the Pediatric Sleep Questionnaire, suggesting sleep-disordered breathing.[36] In some children the disorder is progressive, and death may result from the abnormal ventilatory patterns.[2]

Rett syndrome
Rett syndrome is a genetic disorder caused by a mutation in the MECP2 gene on the X chromosome that affects women. Clinical features include, after a period of normal development, developmental plateauing, then regression, decreased head growth, seizures, autistic features, stereotypical hand movements with eventual loss of purposeful hand function, and expressive language. Breathing disturbances are a characteristic feature of Rett syndrome, which may include episodes of apnea, irregular breathing, and hyperventilation. They are more frequent during wakefulness than during sleep and may involve alternating episodes of hypoventilation and irregular hyperventilation.[37] Research in mouse models suggests areas in the ventrolateral

medulla and pons contribute to the breathing disturbances seen in Rett syndrome.[37]

SUMMARY

Control of breathing in children varies with age and sleep state. There is overlap between central hypoventilation, autonomic dysfunction, and hypothalamic dysfunction in some rare disorders of central hypoventilation (CCHS and ROHHAD). Other disorders that typically present in childhood also include central hypoventilation and disordered ventilatory responses. Please refer to **Table 2** that summarizes the sleep and breathing abnormalities in disorders affecting ventilation. These disorders illustrate the complex interactions of the brain, respiratory muscles, and sleep state and how abnormalities in these areas can significantly alter breathing patterns in sleep and wakefulness. An awareness of these disorders is key to identifying and treating children with abnormal control of breathing. An understanding of the unique relationship between control of breathing and sleep state (NREM vs REM vs wake) is key to the accurate evaluation and treatment of these rare disorders.

CLINICS CARE POINTS

- Hypoventilation is rare in children and requires clinical investigation into cause.
- In the absence of cardiac, pulmonary, or neurologic disease, disorders of central hypoventilation should be considered.
- Hypoventilation in NREM sleep is a key clinical feature of disorders of central hypoventilation; this contrasts with OSA, which is often worse in REM sleep and differs from hypoventilation secondary to neuromuscular disease, which typically occurs first during REM sleep.
- PSG can uncover abnormalities that play a key role in the diagnosis of these rare disorders.

DISCLOSURE

Drs J.M. Baughn and C.A. Matarese have no commercial or financial conflicts of interest and no funding sources.

REFERENCES

1. Principles and Practice of Sleep Medicine, 4th Edition. Kryger MH, Roth T, Dement WC, Editors. Elsevier/Saunders; Philadelphia(PA): 2005.
2. Lesser DJ, Ward SL, Kun SS, et al. Congenital hypoventilation syndromes. Semin Respir Crit Care Med 2009;30(3):339–47.
3. Cielo C, Marcus CL. Central hypoventilation syndromes. Sleep Med Clin 2014;9(1):105–18.
4. Martin RJ, Abu-Shaweesh JM. Control of breathing and neonatal apnea. Biol Neonate 2005;87(4): 288–95.
5. St Louis EK, Jinnur P, McCarter SJ, et al. Chiari 1 malformation presenting as central sleep apnea during pregnancy: a case report, treatment considerations, and review of the literature. Front Neurol 2014;5:195.
6. Fukushi I, Yokota S, Okada Y. The role of the hypothalamus in modulation of respiration. Respir Physiol Neurobiol 2019;265:172–9.
7. Katz ES, Marcus CL, White DP. Influence of airway pressure on genioglossus activity during sleep in normal children. Am J Respir Crit Care Med 2006; 173(8):902–9.
8. Horner RL, Bradley TD. Update in sleep and control of ventilation 2006. Am J Respir Crit Care Med 2007; 175(5):426–31.
9. Givan DC. Physiology of breathing and related pathological processes in infants. Semin Pediatr Neurol 2003;10(4):271–80.
10. Khan A, Qurashi M, Kwiatkowski K, et al. Measurement of the CO2 apneic threshold in newborn infants: possible relevance for periodic breathing and apnea. J Appl Physiol (1985) 2005;98(4): 1171–6.
11. Travers CP, Abman SH, Carlo WA. Control of breathing in preterm infants. Neonatal ICU and beyond. Am J Respir Crit Care Med 2018;197(12):1518–20.
12. Berry RB, Quan SF, Abreu AR, et al. The AASM MAnual for the scoring of sleep and associated events: rules, terminology, and technical specifications. Darien (IL): American Academy of Sleep Medicine; 2020.
13. Medicine AAoS. International classification of sleep disorders, 3rd edition. American Academy of Sleep Medicine; 2014.
14. Carroll MS, Patwari PP, Weese-Mayer DE. Carbon dioxide chemoreception and hypoventilation syndromes with autonomic dysregulation. J Appl Physiol 2010;108(4):979–88.
15. Amiel J, Laudier B, Attié-Bitach T, et al. Polyalanine expansion and frameshift mutations of the paired-like homeobox gene PHOX2B in congenital central hypoventilation syndrome. Nat Genet 2003;33(4): 459–61.
16. Weese-Mayer DE, Berry-Kravis EM, Ceccherini I, et al. An official ATS clinical policy statement: congenital central hypoventilation syndrome: genetic basis, diagnosis, and management. Am J Respir Crit Care Med 2010;181(6):626–44.
17. Balakrishnan K, Perez IA, Keens TG, et al. Hirschsprung disease and other gastrointestinal motility disorders in patients with CCHS. Eur J Pediatr 2021;180(2):469–73.
18. Laifman E, Keens TG, Bar-Cohen Y, et al. Life-threatening cardiac arrhythmias in congenital central hypoventilation syndrome. Eur J Pediatr 2020;179(5): 821–5.
19. Ize-Ludlow D, Gray JA, Sperling MA, et al. Rapid-onset obesity with hypothalamic dysfunction, hypoventilation, and autonomic dysregulation presenting in childhood. Pediatrics 2007;120(1):e179–88.
20. Katz ES, McGrath S, Marcus CL. Late-onset central hypoventilation with hypothalamic dysfunction: a distinct clinical syndrome. Pediatr Pulmonol 2000; 29(1):62–8.
21. Bougneres P, Pantalone L, Linglart A, et al. Endocrine manifestations of the rapid-onset obesity with hypoventilation, hypothalamic, autonomic dysregulation, and neural tumor syndrome in childhood. J Clin Endocrinol Metab 2008;93(10):3971–80.
22. Harvengt J, Gernay C, Mastouri M, et al. ROHHAD(-NET) syndrome: systematic review of the clinical timeline and recommendations for diagnosis and prognosis. J Clin Endocrinol Metab 2020;105(7): dgaa247.

23. Rand CM, Patwari PP, Rodikova EA, et al. Rapid-onset obesity with hypothalamic dysfunction, hypoventilation, and autonomic dysregulation: analysis of hypothalamic and autonomic candidate genes. Pediatr Res 2011;70(4):375–8.

24. Urquhart DS, Gulliver T, Williams G, et al. Central sleep-disordered breathing and the effects of oxygen therapy in infants with Prader-Willi syndrome. Arch Dis Child 2013;98(8):592–5.

25. Gillett ES, Perez IA. Disorders of sleep and ventilatory control in prader-willi syndrome. Diseases 2016;4(3):23.

26. Katz-Salamon M, Lindgren AC, Cohen G. The effect of growth hormone on sleep-related cardio-respiratory control in Prader-Willi syndrome. Acta Paediatr 2012;101(6):643–8.

27. Zanella S, Tauber M, Muscatelli F. Breathing deficits of the Prader-Willi syndrome. Respir Physiol Neurobiol 2009;168(1–2):119–24.

28. Gold-von Simson G, Axelrod FB. Familial dysautonomia: update and recent advances. Curr Probl Pediatr Adolesc Health Care 2006;36(6):218–37.

29. Ferré Á, Poca MA, de la Calzada MD, et al. Sleep-related breathing disorders in Chiari malformation type 1: a prospective study of 90 patients. Sleep 2017;40(6):1–5.

30. Bhangoo R, Sgouros S, Walsh AR, et al. Hindbrain-hernia-related syringomyelia without syringobulbia, complicated by permanent nocturnal central hypoventilation requiring non-invasive ventilation. Childs Nerv Syst 2006;22(2):113–6.

31. Mogayzel PJ Jr, Carroll JL, Loughlin GM, et al. Sleep-disordered breathing in children with achondroplasia. J Pediatr 1998;132(4):667–71.

32. Stokes DC, Phillips JA, Leonard CO, et al. Respiratory complications of achondroplasia. J Pediatr 1983;102(4):534–41.

33. Ednick M, Tinkle BT, Phromchairak J, et al. Sleep-related respiratory abnormalities and arousal pattern in achondroplasia during early infancy. J Pediatr 2009;155(4):510–5.

34. Trotter TL, Hall JG. Health supervision for children with achondroplasia. Pediatrics 2005;116(3):771–83.

35. Mallepally AR, Karthik Y, Ansari N, et al. Reversible central hypoventilation syndrome in basilar invagination. World Neurosurg 2019;131:120–5.

36. Kamdar BB, Nandkumar P, Krishnan V, et al. Self-reported sleep and breathing disturbances in Joubert syndrome. Pediatr Neurol 2011;45(6):395–9.

37. Ramirez JM, Ward CS, Neul JL. Breathing challenges in Rett syndrome: lessons learned from humans and animal models. Respir Physiol Neurobiol 2013;189(2):280–7.

What's New in Pediatric Obstructive Sleep Apnea?

Christopher M. Cielo, DO, MSTR*, Ignacio E. Tapia, MD, MSTR

KEYWORDS

- Obstructive sleep apnea • Children • Pediatric

KEY POINTS

- Drug-induced sleep endoscopy can be used to identify the site of upper airway obstruction in patients with obstructive sleep apnea (OSA), including those with Down syndrome.
- Home sleep apnea testing for the evaluation of OSA in children is feasible; larger clinical trials comparing to polysomnography including patient-centered outcomes are needed to support implementation.
- Hypoglossal nerve stimulation may provide an additional treatment option for adolescents with Down syndrome who have moderate-severe refractory OSA.
- There are several treatment options that have been shown to be effective in infants with OSA, including CPAP, high-flow nasal cannula, and low-flow oxygen.

INTRODUCTION

Obstructive sleep apnea (OSA) is common children, and continues to be the focus of recent research, including the evaluation and management of OSA in children, and the association between OSA and other comorbidities in childhood. Although the evaluation of OSA has traditionally involved office-based clinical assessment and polysomnography, there is a demand for more family-focused evaluation and novel diagnostic approaches, especially given challenges during the coronavirus disease 2019 (COVID-19) pandemic. Through partnerships with airway surgeons, drug-induced sleep endoscopy is increasingly being used clinically in children with Down syndrome and other comorbidities in surgical planning. In addition, multiple studies have investigated the feasibility and accuracy of out-of laboratory testing for the evaluation of OSA in children. These and other novel diagnostics could lead to an expansion of OSA testing and a more targeted approach to treatment. Several studies have examined the association between OSA and other comorbidities during childhood, including several that have assessed the association between early lower respiratory tract illnesses and OSA. These studies contribute to the existing literature about the overall impact of OSA on childhood health. Therapeutic options for OSA in children remain limited. Hypoglossal nerve stimulation has been shown to be an effective therapy for OSA in adults, and recent studies have examined its utility in children with Down syndrome. Positive airway pressure (PAP) has been a mainstay of OSA treatment, but adherence is often suboptimal. Several recent studies have assessed factors associated with adherence, and findings could lead to more effective use of PAP in children with OSA. Infants are a challenging age to treat for OSA, with fewer therapeutic options than for older children and adults. Several recent studies have examined the utility of various treatment approaches that may provide options to clinicians caring for these young patients.

EVALUATION OF OBSTRUCTIVE SLEEP APNEA IN CHILDREN
Drug-Induced Sleep Endoscopy

Drug-induced sleep endoscopy (DISE) is a flexible fiberoptic endoscopy performed under sedation

Division of Pulmonary and Sleep Medicine, Children's Hospital of Philadelphia, Perelman School of Medicine, University of Pennsylvania, Philadelphia, PA, USA
* Corresponding author. Hub For Clinical Collaboration, Children's Hospital of Philadelphia, 3501 Civic Center Boulevard, Philadelphia, PA 19104.
E-mail address: cieloc@chop.edu

Sleep Med Clin 18 (2023) 173–181
https://doi.org/10.1016/j.jsmc.2023.02.002
1556-407X/23/© 2023 Elsevier Inc. All rights reserved.

while the patient is breathing spontaneously to determine, in a dynamic view, sites of upper airway obstruction to inform the utility or indication of surgical interventions (**Fig. 1**). DISE is gaining more importance in pediatrics, as OSA, particularly in children with obesity and other comorbidities, does not completely resolve after adenotonsillectomy. The American Academy of Otolaryngology-Head and Neck Surgery (AAO-HNS) recently published an expert consensus statement on pediatric DISE to clarify utility and indications, controversies of the procedure, and propose research directions. [1] The authors identified 26 expert statements, a summary of which is provided:

- Polysomnography is recommended prior to DISE to confirm presence and severity of OSA.
- DISE at the time of adenotonsillectomy is limited in children with OSA and adenotonsillar hypertrophy not at risk for persistent OSA.
- The level of sedation during pediatric DISE should be titrated to audible snoring, an obstructive breathing pattern, or both while allowing for flexible endoscopy without patient reactivity or awakening.
- The following parameters should be observed and documented for each anatomic level: (a) site, (b) pattern or shape, and (c) severity of obstruction.
- The following anatomic sites should be assessed and documented: nasal airway (including nasal cavities, nasopharynx), palate/velum, pharyngeal airway (including lateral oropharyngeal wall and tongue base), and supraglottic larynx.
- Children with OSA undergoing DISE may be discharged the same day.

Raposo and colleagues described 56 children with OSA who underwent DISE before upper airway surgery. Of these, 23 were surgically naïve, and 33 had undergone adenotonsillectomy. The authors found out that the sites of obstruction differed between the 2 groups. Surgically naïve children's common sites of obstruction were related to adenotonsillar hypertrophy, while supraglottis and tongue-based obstructions were common sites of upper airway collapse in those with persistent OSA. [2] Importantly, the obstructive apnea hypopnea index did not correlate with DISE results. This may have been related to the relatively small sample size. Hyzer and colleagues reported one of the largest pediatric DISE cohorts (N = 317) of surgically naïve children including a small group of children with Down syndrome (N = 23). [3] The latter, compared to children without Down syndrome, demonstrated worse overall obstruction, with a mean Sleep Endoscopy Rating Scale total score of 5.6 (95% confidence interval [CI], 4.9–6.2) versus 4.8 (95% CI, 4.4–5.1; Cohen d, 0.46). Children with Down syndrome had more multilevel obstruction, including tonsillar (65 vs 54%), tongue-based (26 vs 12%), and arytenoid obstruction (35 vs 6%). Maris and colleagues had reported comparable results in a cohort of 41 children with Down syndrome. [4] Future randomized controlled trials evaluating the use of DISE in children with and without comorbidities are needed.

Home Sleep Apnea Testing

With the growing awareness of OSA in children and the paucity of facilities to evaluate for sleep-disordered breathing, there has been a growth in studies assessing the feasibility and accuracy of emerging technologies beyond in-laboratory polysomnography (PSG) in children, particularly as

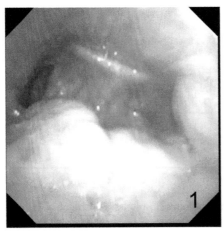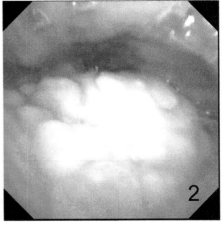

Fig. 1. In patients with obstructive sleep apnea, drug-induced sleep endoscopic findings of obstruction at the level of the epiglottis (*image 1*) and base of tongue (*image 2*). (Images courtesy of Ryan Borek, MD.)

sleep laboratories were less available during the COVID-19 pandemic.

One study compared the success rate of shifting children from in-laboratory PSG to type III home respiratory polygraphy (HRP) in the first 3 months of the COVID-19 pandemic in the United Kingdom. 5 Of the 96 children who underwent HRP, median (IQR) age 5 (2–9) years old, only 56% had greater than 4 hours of interpretable sleep data available. Children under the age of 5 and those with autism spectrum disorder or attention deficit hyperactivity disorder had the lowest success rate. Importantly, the study design included a home-based setup, and the most common signal that failed was the chest and abdominal bands. Most families surveyed felt that HRP could be beneficial, although some expressed concern about setting up the equipment at home.

Another study that used a home-based setup of type III HSAT with overnight video support in children showed a higher rate of success. 6 One hundred children aged 3 to 11 years were randomized to in-laboratory PSG or HSAT, and feasibility, family preference, and sleep parameters were compared. Of the 50 children randomized to HSAT, 46% had at least 70% valid data collected during the study. There were no differences in respiratory parameters for the group randomized to HSAT compared with PSG, but the children who underwent HSAT spent more time in bed and appeared to be sleeping significantly more than those studied in the sleep laboratory.

A third recently published study based in Australia directly compared in-laboratory PSG with type II HSAT that included electroencephalogram (EEG). In this study, 81 children over 5 years old had HSAT conducted simultaneously with PSG in the sleep laboratory, and another 47 children completed HSAT at home on a night separate from their PSG. 7 All HSAT studies were considered acceptable for diagnostic purposes, and there was a high degree of diagnostic agreement between the 2 tests, with HSAT having a 6.6% false-positive rate for OSA diagnosis and a 3% false negative rate compared with in-laboratory PSG.

Although the results of these and other previously published studies have shown promise for the feasibility and accuracy of HSAT for the evaluation of OSA in children, most include cohorts that are limited in size, age range, racial and ethnic diversity, and inclusion of medically complex children. Larger clinical trials that evaluate the impact of HSAT on therapeutic decision making and include family-centered outcomes will be needed before these tests can be considered a true alternative to PSG for most children.

ASSOCIATION BETWEEN PEDIATRIC OBSTRUCTIVE SLEEP APNEA AND OTHER COMORBIDITIES

Several recent studies have examined the relationship between OSA and other comorbidities in children, including dyslipidemia, insulin resistance, obesity, inflammation, and changes in the oral microbiome. [8–11] In addition, several studies have examined the relationship of lower respiratory tract illnesses (LRTI) early in life with OSA.

A recent study by Gutierrez and colleagues used the Boston Birth Cohort to evaluate the association between LRTI in the first 2 years of life and OSA by age 5. [12] Utilizing prospectively collected data in over 3000 children, an adjusted hazard ratio of 1.53 was found for incident OSA during the first 5 years of life, and there was a twofold increase in the odds of OSA among children hospitalized for bronchiolitis by age 2. These same associations were not seen for LRTI between 2 and 5 years of age.

A second study by Tsou and colleagues used the Kid's Inpatient Database to compare the outcomes of children hospitalized with bronchiolitis based on their OSA status, including those with and without Down syndrome. [13] Analysis included over 900,000 bronchiolitis admissions for children less than 2 years old, including nearly 9000 admissions for children with Down syndrome. OSA status was associated with an odds ratio of 3.32 for invasive mechanical ventilation during hospitalization compared with no OSA, and in young children with Down syndrome, OSA was also associated with increased noninvasive ventilation and cost of hospitalization. Taken together, these 2 studies suggest a bidirectional association between early LRTI and OSA, which could be exacerbated in high-risk children such as those with Down syndrome.

Overall, this growing body of literature suggests that there are significant associations between OSA and other medical comorbidities in children in addition to neurobehavioral consequences that have previously been described. These and other studies suggest targets for pediatric OSA clinical trials and reinforce the importance of OSA diagnosis and treatment as a part of child health.

PEDIATRIC OBSTRUCTIVE SLEEP APNEA THERAPEUTICS
Treatment of Obstructive Sleep Apnea in Infants/Young Children

Increasingly, OSA is being recognized in high-risk infants, including those with craniofacial conditions, Down syndrome, and other risk factors, [14–16] including the interpretation of polysomnography in these very young patients. [17] However, nonsurgical treatment of OSA in infants remains challenging because of a lack of well-accepted best-practice guidelines and the various underlying causes of OSA in infants. Several recent studies have evaluated different therapies for OSA treatment in these patients (**Table 1**).

The authors' group conducted a retrospective analysis comparing the efficacy, adherence, and parent-reported barriers of continuous positive airway pressure (CPAP) for the treatment of OSA in infants compared with school-age children. [18] The study included 41 infants less than 6 months of age and 109 children 5 to 10 years old who underwent baseline and titrate polysomnography, had PAP adherence data downloaded, and had standardized report of barriers to adherence. The study found that despite infants treated having a greater apnea-hypopnea index (AHI) than school-age children, PAP was highly effective, with a median obstructive apnea-hypopnea index (OAHI) reduction of 92%, and 82% of infants having a residual OAHI less than 5/h on PAP titration. PAP was used by infants on more nights than school-age children (95% vs 83%), and there were no differences in the barriers to adherence. This single-center study reviewed the results of treatment conducted by an experienced interdisciplinary team that included dedicated respiratory therapists, nurses, and psychologists. At centers with more limited resources, treating infants with PAP may be less effective.

An alternative therapy to CPAP for the treatment of OSA in infants is high-flow nasal cannula, which has been used in older children with OSA and infants with bronchopulmonary dysplasia. [19,20] One recent report recently examined the use of heated humidified high-flow nasal cannula (HHHFNC) in 10 infants with OSA. [21] This retrospective study assessed baseline OSA severity and oxyhemoglobin saturation during a nap study in the sleep laboratory, and then titrated HHHFNC between 4 and 8 liters per minute of flow during the second portion of the study to reduce OAHI and normalize oxyhemoglobin saturation. In this cohort, which had a median (interquartile range) age of 48 (46, 52) weeks corrected gestational age, including half with a history of prematurity, baseline OAHI was reduced from 9.1 (5.1, 19.3) events per hour to 0.9 (0, 1.6) events per hour ($P=.005$), with significant reduction in the obstructive apnea index and obstructive hypopnea index and saturation nadir. There were 5 additional patients who required supplemental oxygen in addition to HHHFNC in order to treat OSA effectively.

A second retrospective study used a similar methodology in 22 older infants with OSA who were not candidates for surgical treatment and/or were refractory to CPAP. [22] Patients whose mean (95%

Table 1
Non-surgical therapies for OSA in infants

	Proposed Mechanism	Advantages	Challenges	Reference
CPAP	Pneumatic stent prevents airway collapse	• Established therapy in older children • Titration study can confirm efficacy	• Obtaining appropriate equipment may be challenge for some infants • Some centers may not have expertise/personnel to implement and support families	Cielo et al,[18] 2021
HHHFNC	Maintain nasopharyngeal patency, reduce inspiratory resistance	• Reduced desensitization compared to CPAP • Nasal interfaces for infants widely available	• Equipment and flow rate less standardized • Assessment of airflow on titration PSG may be challenging • Less objective adherence tracking	Kwok et al,[21] 2020; Ignatiuk et al,[22] 2020
Low flow oxygen	Stabilize ventilatory control, prevents desaturation required for scoring some hypopneas	• Widely available • Minimal desensitization needed • Titration PSG can assess efficacy	• Significant residual OSA in many • Less objective adherence tracking	Brockbank et al,[23] 2019

CI) age was 8.1 months (4.6-11.6) underwent a diagnostic PSG and then returned for a titration with the high-flow nasal cannula, where flow was adjusted between 1 and 12 liters per minute. There was a significant reduction in the OAHI from the diagnostic study: 28.9 events per hour (17.6-40.2) to the optimal flow setting: 2.6 events per hour (1.1-4.0). Although HHHFNC setups can be simpler to fit infants than CPAP, adherence cannot be tracked as easily, and flow signals may be difficult to interpret on titration polysomnography, making some respiratory events potentially more difficult to score.

Low-flow supplemental oxygen has also been studied as a potential treatment for OSA in infants. Compared with other modalities, low-flow oxygen has the potential to improve central apnea and periodic breathing and requires a less complex setup that may be more readily available. Brockbank and colleagues performed a single-center retrospective analysis of 59 infants aged 13 plus or minus 12 weeks old who had a diagnostic PSG and then repeated PSG with nasal cannula in place, typically one-eighth to one-fourth liter per minute. [23] Although there was a significant reduction in the OAHI (from 19.7 $\pm$ 13.0 events/h to 10.6 $\pm$ 11.7 events/h) and overall AHI, there was no change in the obstructive apnea index. This effect was likely due at least in part to reduced scoring of both central apneas and obstructive hypopneas because of a lack of desaturation associated with the use of supplemental oxygen. There were not significant adverse effects in terms of alveolar ventilation, but OAHI failed to normalize in many infants. Although low-flow supplemental oxygen may not be able to definitively treat obstructive apnea in infants, it is a widely available therapy that could offer a safe and effective treatment to a selected group of infants.

Although taken together, these studies suggest that there are multiple effective treatment options for infants with OSA, outcomes are primarily restricted to PSG data, and no long-term outcome studies are available. Larger, longitudinal studies of infants with OSA are needed, as are clinical trials comparing surgical and nonsurgical approaches to OSA in these young patients.

Positive Airway Pressure Adherence

PAP remains a mainstay of OSA therapy in adults and children, but adherence to PAP remains a challenge. Several recent studies have examined factors associated with adherence to PAP in children, taking advantage of objective electronic usage data to assess factors associated with adherence, which could eventually lead to targeted approaches to improve the efficacy of PAP.

Weiss and colleagues retrospectively analyzed cloud-based PAP data in 250 diverse children with OSA aged 1 month to 18 years during a relatively short average period of 65 days. [24] Subgroups based on PAP tolerance (average hours of PAP use on days used) and consistency of PAP use (percentage of days used) were created using cluster analysis. The cohort was then classified into 5 clusters: A-best PAP tolerance and consistent use, B- acceptable PAP tolerance and consistent use, C- poor tolerance to PAP therapy and consistent use, D-acceptable PAP tolerance and inconsistent use, and finally E—poor PAP tolerance and inconsistent use. Forty-four percent of the children were grouped in clusters A and B. Investigators proposed an algorithm targeting interventions based on clustering, toward modifiable characteristics such as weight loss, interface optimization, and behavioral desensitization, among others. This personalized clustering is a commendable example of the use of telemonitoring to improve adherence at a population level. Future prospective studies including socio-ecological factors and longer periods of data download are needed. [25]

Another study prospectively evaluated factors associated with adherence to PAP in a cohort of obese youth with newly diagnosed OSA. [26] Twelve months after PAP initiation, objective machine downloads were assessed for usage, and participants completed a questionnaire assessing knowledge and understanding of PAP, supports, attitudes, and experiences with PAP and its social impact. Eleven (79%) of the 14 participants who completed the 12-month follow-up were adherent (mean PAP use of greater than 4 hours per night). All parents surveyed expected their child to feel better with PAP use, and 71.4% of youth reported sleeping better when PAP is used; however, 78.6% reported having adverse effects from PAP. With the small sample size, the only baseline characteristic associated with increased adherence was lower oxyhemoglobin saturation nadir on diagnostic polysomnogram. Interestingly, the majority of both children and parents reported that the child (including some as young as 8 years old) were in charge of their PAP usage. Although larger studies are clearly needed to further examine these trends, approaches to improve adherence could include targeted strategies that partner parent and child early on to identify barriers and make adjustments.

Although these studies and others offer insight into potential parent/child perception and barriers to PAP use, larger datasets with objective, longitudinal PAP usage data, and qualitative and implementation research data are needed to better understand factors associated with adherence to help define reasonable expectations for insurance and durable medical equipment companies. In addition, pediatric-focused clinical trials are needed to determine effective interventions to improve adherence. One recent meta-analysis found that adequate family support was associated with improved adherence,[27] and additional factors could include the type of support available from the medical team prescribing the PAP for these patients who often have significant additional comorbidities.

Hypoglossal Nerve Stimulation

Hypoglossal nerve (HGN) stimulation is a treatment available clinically for moderate-severe OSA in adults where a surgically implanted pulse generator prevents tongue-based airway collapse by electrical stimulation of the hypoglossal nerve. Previous studies have shown a therapy response in 63% to 69% of adults, but HGN has not previously been evaluated in younger patients.

A recently completed single-group clinical trial evaluated the safety and efficacy of HGN in adolescents with Down syndrome who had persistent OSA after adenotonsillectomy.[28] The multicenter study enrolled 42 youth at 5 academic centers, where they underwent surgical implantation of the HGN device and had 1 year of follow-up, with serial PSG, questionnaires, and safety assessments. From a median (range) baseline OAHI of 22.0 events per hour (9.7), there was a reduction of 12.2 events per hour (12.7) at 12-month assessment. Twenty-seven of 41 participants (65.9%) had at least a 50% reduction in AHI. However, significant residual OSA was common, with only 14 of 41 participants (34.1%) having a final AHI less than 5 events per hour. There was a significant reduction in the Epworth Sleepiness scale and significant improvement in the OSA-18 score from baseline to endpoint. HGN was overall well tolerated, with 95.2% of participants using the device for more than 4 hours per night for 70% of nights; 11.9% of participants reported temporary tongue or oral discomfort, and other complications included rash, ulcers, and cellulitis. Five participants (11.9%) required readmission, and 2 patients (4.8%) required reoperation; 1 participant developed postobstructive central hypoventilation. Youth with circumferential palatal collapse, obesity, and with an apnea hypopnea index of greater than 50 events per hour were not eligible to undergo HGN in the trial. In children, HGN has only been studied in youth 10 to 21 years old with Down syndrome and is not currently available for clinical care. A second trial is underway in a similar age range of youth with Down syndrome that will examine neurocognitive outcomes following HGN.

FUTURE DIRECTIONS

There has been a significant expansion in studies examining the evaluation and management of OSA in children, as well as the association between OSA and other medical comorbidities. However, there have been fewer changes in the clinical care of children with OSA. To significantly reduce the delays to diagnosis of OSA and improve OSA-associated morbidity, additional work is needed in several key areas

Expand the Capacity for Obstructive Sleep Apnea Evaluation in Children

If children with OSA cannot be identified, they cannot be referred for the appropriate treatment. Both medical technology and consumer wearables are advancing faster than the limited number of researchers in this area can study them. Therefore, partnerships between manufacturers, clinicians, researchers, and families are needed during the development, implementation, and validation phases to develop the best OSA evaluation technology for infants, children, and adolescents, and ensure equipment is safe and child-friendly.

To support this development, larger pediatric trials will be needed to provide adequate evidence to support implementation beyond the research setting. These studies should include family-centered outcomes and real-world medical decision making, which have been barriers to scaling up previous small studies. An ongoing clinical trial is comparing the validity of home respiratory polygraphy with polysomnography in a large cohort of children age 2 to 14 years referred for evaluation of OSA.[29] This multicenter randomized cross-over trial will assess medical decision making and cost in addition to accuracy of home respiratory polygraphy to PSG. The authors' group will be conducting a large clinical trial comparing the accuracy, preference, and impact on therapeutic decision making between type II home sleep apnea testing and in-laboratory PSG (**Fig. 2**). In addition, a pipeline must be developed to evaluate emerging technologies that assess sleep and OSA in children, including machine-learning tools to improve efficiency in sleep testing.

Increase Inclusivity in Pediatric Obstructive Sleep Apnea Studies

To develop diagnostics and therapeutics that will benefit all children, studies including clinical trials must include better representation from children from all races and ethnicity, as well as participants with limited English proficiency. In addition, children with underlying medical and developmental

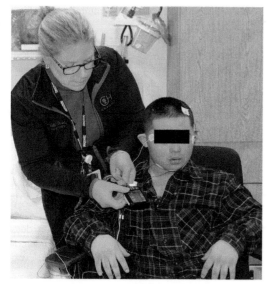

Fig. 2. Sleep technologist setting up an adolescent with Down syndrome for a level II home sleep apnea test.

conditions must be included in these studies to ensure that this substantial portion of the children we care for are not denied access to the potential benefits of study participation or the therapies when they become available for clinical use.

BETTER UNDERSTAND THE HISTORY OF OBSTRUCTIVE SLEEP APNEA ACROSS THE SPECTRUM OF CHILDHOOD

Studies of pediatric OSA have shown improvement in some children after a period of watchful waiting, [30] and there is evidence that there may be significant changes in the apnea hypopnea index with growth, particularly in infants. [31] However, the natural history of OSA in childhood is poorly understood throughout the pediatric age spectrum. Longitudinal studies, ideally including birth cohorts, could help better define risk factors for OSA at different stages of childhood and understand relationship between pediatric and adult OSA.

Identify Key Outcome Variables for Pediatric Obstructive Sleep Apnea Trials

Although numerous neurobehavioral, metabolic, and cardiovascular outcomes have been evaluated in studies of pediatric OSA, [32–34] an established set of outcome variables beyond polysomnographic metrics could be useful as therapeutic targets, ideally spanning the pediatric age spectrum. Big data approaches could help establish such endpoints and provide a better understanding of the impact of OSA on overall child

health, both for otherwise healthy children and those with underlying comorbidities.

Improve and Expand the Treatment Options for Children with Obstructive Sleep Apnea

In most cases, treatment options remain limited to adenotonsillectomy and CPAP, with other therapies having limited efficacy or only being available to small groups of patients. Partnerships are needed with colleagues in surgical disciplines and with industry to develop additional safe, effective treatments for OSA in children across the age spectrum and establish precision-medicine tools to establish the best treatment for each patient. This includes improved models of CPAP adherence, identifying optimal surgical candidates, and increasing pediatric access to therapies available for adults.

Expand the Medical Providers Who Evaluate and Manage Obstructive Sleep Apnea in Children

There are insufficient pediatric sleep medicine physicians to direct the management of all children with OSA. Improved models of partnering with colleagues to screen for OSA in the community and specialty care clinics and with surgical colleagues to ensure best practices in the management of OSA are needed. In addition, efforts are needed to expand the pipeline of multidisciplinary and interdisciplinary providers who do have training in pediatric sleep medicine. Finally, funding is needed for investigators with training, expertise, and interest in improving the evaluation and management of OSA in children spanning the spectrum of basic, translational, and clinical research.

CLINICS CARE POINTS

- Consider drug-induced sleep endoscopy in children with persistent OSA after adenotonsillectomy to provide information about planning additional surgery.
- Home sleep apnea testing is currently not recommended for the clinical evaluation of OSA in children.
- For infants with OSA, consider treatment with CPAP, high-flow nasal cannula, or low-flow nasal cannula oxygen depending on OSA severity, patient factors, and support staff.
- Involve children and caregivers in CPAP initiation to improve adherence and identify potential challenges early in the process.

FUNDING

Cielo and Tapia: NIH R61 HL162839.

REFERENCES

1. Baldassari CM, Lam DJ, Ishman SL, et al. Expert consensus statement: pediatric drug-induced sleep endoscopy. Otolaryngol Head Neck Surg 2021; 165(4):578–91.

2. Raposo D, Menezes M, Rito J, et al. Drug-induced sleep endoscopy in pediatric obstructive sleep apnea. Otolaryngol Head Neck Surg 2021;164(2): 414–21.

3. Hyzer JM, Milczuk HA, Macarthur CJ, et al. Drug-induced sleep endoscopy findings in children with obstructive sleep apnea with vs without obesity or Down syndrome. JAMA Otolaryngol Head Neck Surg 2021;147(2):175–81.

4. Maris M, Verhulst S, Saldien V, et al. Drug-induced sedation endoscopy in surgically naive children with Down syndrome and obstructive sleep apnea. Sleep Med 2016;24:63–70.

5. Jones S, Hanwell R, Chowdhury T, et al. Feasibility and parental perception of home sleep studies during COVID-19: a tertiary sleep centre experience. Arch Dis Child 2022;107(2):189–91.

6. Green A, Nagel N, Kemer L, et al. Comparing in-lab full polysomnography for diagnosing sleep apnea in children to home sleep apnea tests (HSAT) with an online video attending technician. Sleep Biol Rhythms 2022;1–5.

7. Withers A, Maul J, Rosenheim E, et al. Comparison of home ambulatory type 2 polysomnography with a portable monitoring device and in-laboratory type 1 polysomnography for the diagnosis of obstructive sleep apnea in children. J Clin Sleep Med 2022;18(2):393–402.

8. Bhatt SP, Guleria R, Kabra SK. Metabolic alterations and systemic inflammation in overweight/obese children with obstructive sleep apnea. PLoS One 2021; 16(6):e0252353.

9. Kang EK, Jang MJ, Kim KD, et al. The association of obstructive sleep apnea with dyslipidemia in Korean children and adolescents: a single-center, cross-sectional study. J Clin Sleep Med 2021;17(8): 1599–605.

10. Siriwat R, Wang L, Shah V, et al. Obstructive sleep apnea and insulin resistance in children with obesity. J Clin Sleep Med 2020;16(7):1081–90.

11. Xu H, Li X, Zheng X, et al. Pediatric obstructive sleep apnea is associated with changes in the oral microbiome and urinary metabolomics profile: a pilot study. J Clin Sleep Med 2018;14(9):1559–67.

12. Gutierrez MJ, Nino G, Landeo-Gutierrez JS, et al. Lower respiratory tract infections in early life are associated with obstructive sleep apnea diagnosis during childhood in a large birth cohort. Sleep 2021;44(12).

13. Tsou PY, Cielo CM, Xanthopoulos MS, et al. The impact of obstructive sleep apnea on bronchiolitis severity in children with Down syndrome. Sleep Med 2021;83:188–95.

14. Waters KA, Castro C, Chawla J. The spectrum of obstructive sleep apnea in infants and children with Down Syndrome. Int J Pediatr Otorhinolaryngol 2019;129:109763.

15. Maclean JE, Fitzsimons D, Fitzgerald DA, et al. The spectrum of sleep-disordered breathing symptoms and respiratory events in infants with cleft lip and/or palate. Arch Dis Child 2012; 97(12):1058–63.

16. Huang YS, Hsu JF, Paiva T, et al. Sleep-disordered breathing, craniofacial development, and neurodevelopment in premature infants: a 2-year follow-up study. Sleep Med 2019;60:20–5.

17. Daftary AS, Jalou HE, Shively L, et al. Polysomnography reference values in healthy Newborns. J Clin Sleep Med 2019;15(3):437–43.

18. Cielo CM, Hernandez P, Ciampaglia AM, et al. Positive airway pressure for the treatment of obstructive sleep apnea syndrome in infants. Chest 2021; 159(2):810–7.

19. Shetty S, Hickey A, Rafferty GF, et al. Work of breathing during CPAP and heated humidified high-flow nasal cannula. Arch Dis Child Fetal Neonatal Ed 2016;101(5):F404–7.

20. McGinley B, Halbower A, Schwartz AR, et al. Effect of a high-flow open nasal cannula system on obstructive sleep apnea in children. Pediatrics 2009;124(1):179–88.

21. Kwok KL, Lau MY, Leung SY, et al. Use of heated humidified high flow nasal cannula for obstructive sleep apnea in infants. Sleep Med 2020;74:332–7.

22. Ignatiuk D, Schaer B, McGinley B. High flow nasal cannula treatment for obstructive sleep apnea in infants and young children. Pediatr Pulmonol 2020; 55(10):2791–8.

23. Brockbank J, Astudillo CL, Che D, et al. Supplemental oxygen for treatment of infants with obstructive sleep apnea. J Clin Sleep Med 2019;15(8):1115–23.

24. Weiss MR, Allen ML, Landeo-Gutierrez JS, et al. Defining the patterns of PAP adherence in pediatric obstructive sleep apnea: a clustering analysis using real-world data. J Clin Sleep Med 2021;17(5): 1005–13.

25. Xanthopoulos MS, Williamson AA, Tapia IE. Positive airway pressure for the treatment of the childhood obstructive sleep apnea syndrome. Pediatr Pulmonol 2022;57(8):1897–903.

26. Katz SL, Kirk VG, MacLean JE, et al. Factors related to positive airway pressure therapy adherence in children with obesity and sleep-disordered breathing. J Clin Sleep Med 2020;16(5):733–41.

27. Sawunyavisuth B, Ngamjarus C, Sawanyawisuth K. Any effective intervention to improve CPAP adherence in children with obstructive sleep apnea: a Systematic Review. Glob Pediatr Health 2021;8. 2333794X211019884.

28. Yu PK, Stenerson M, Ishman SL, et al. Evaluation of upper airway stimulation for adolescents with Down syndrome and obstructive sleep apnea. JAMA Otolaryngol Head Neck Surg 2022;148(6):522–8.

29. Oceja E, Rodriguez P, Jurado MJ, et al. Validity and cost-Effectiveness of pediatric home respiratory polygraphy for the diagnosis of obstructive sleep apnea in children: Rationale, study design, and methodology. Methods Protoc 2021;4(1).

30. Marcus CL, Moore RH, Rosen CL, et al. A randomized trial of adenotonsillectomy for childhood sleep apnea. N Engl J Med 2013;368(25):2366–76.

31. Brockmann PE, Poets A, Poets CF. Reference values for respiratory events in overnight polygraphy from infants aged 1 and 3months. Sleep Med 2013; 14(12):1323–7.

32. Xanthopoulos MS, Gallagher PR, Berkowitz RI, et al. Neurobehavioral functioning in adolescents with and without obesity and obstructive sleep apnea. Sleep 2015;38(3):401–10.

33. Gozal D, Crabtree VM, Sans Capdevila O, et al. C-reactive protein, obstructive sleep apnea, and cognitive dysfunction in school-aged children. Am J Respir Crit Care Med 2007;176(2):188–93.

34. Amin R, Somers VK, McConnell K, et al. Activity-adjusted 24-hour ambulatory blood pressure and cardiac remodeling in children with sleep disordered breathing. Hypertension 2008;51(1):84–91.

Narcolepsy and Idiopathic Hypersomnia

Margaret Blattner, MD, PhD[a], Kiran Maski, MD, MPH[b,*]

KEYWORDS

- Pediatric • Narcolepsy • Hypersomnia • MSLT

KEY POINTS

- Central disorders of hypersomnolence, including narcolepsy type1 and 2 and idiopathic hypersomnia, often have onset in childhood or adolescence but diagnosis is commonly delayed. Recognition of symptoms of these disorders will improve timeliness and accuracy of diagnoses.
- A clinical history including sleep timing, sleep duration, naps, and associated sleep symptoms may help differentiate sleep disorders.
- An overnight polysomnogram (PSG) and daytime multiple sleep latency testing (MSLT) or cerebrospinal fluid orexin testing is the gold standard for narcolepsy type 1; however, this PSG/MSLT sleep study testing has poor reliability in adults with narcolepsy type 2 and idiopathic hypersomnia.
- Insufficient sleep, circadian rhythm disorders, and certain medications may contribute to false-positive results on the multiple sleep latency test.
- There is no cure for narcolepsy or idiopathic hypersomnia; behavioral and pharmacologic treatments aim to reduce sleepiness and cataplexy and improve function.

INTRODUCTION

Narcolepsy types 1 and 2 and idiopathic hypersomnia are debilitating primary central nervous system disorders of hypersomnolence characterized by daytime sleepiness and/or excessive sleep need. Although the pathophysiology of narcolepsy type 2 and idiopathic hypersomnia has not been elucidated, narcolepsy type 1 develops due to a presumed autoimmune-mediated loss of orexin neurons in the lateral hypothalamus. These disorders often have onset in childhood or adolescence, and the presentation of sleepiness and cataplexy (a symptom of narcolepsy type 1) in children can manifest differently than in adults. The goal of this review is to describe a clinical approach, diagnostic evaluation, and management of children and adolescents with excessive daytime sleepiness due narcolepsy types 1 and 2, and idiopathic hypersomnia.

Initial Approach to the Sleepy Child/Adolescent

The International Classification of Sleep Disorders, version 3 (ICSD3) defines hypersomnolence as the irrepressible need to sleep or episodes of daytime sleepiness.[1] The first challenge of identifying central disorders of hypersomnolence in children and adolescents is evaluating the degree and pattern of excessive daytime sleepiness. The experience and description of sleepiness are subjective but most report falling asleep or feeling drowsy in passive situations (ie, reading, in classroom lecture, being driven, waiting patiently) and more rarely sudden sleep attacks. Sleepiness in children may manifest differently than in adults. Sleepy children may have hyperactivity, irritability, inattention, or emotional lability.[2,3] The Epworth Sleepiness Scale for Children and Adolescents (ESS-CHAD)[4] or the Pediatric Daytime Sleepiness Scale

[a] Department of Neurology, Beth Israel Deaconess Medical Center, Harvard Medical School, 330 Brookline Avenue, Boston, MA 02215, USA; [b] Department of Neurology, Boston Children's Hospital, Harvard Medical School, 300 Longwood Avenue, BCH3443, Boston, MA 02115, USA
* Corresponding author.
E-mail address: Kiran.maski@childrens.harvard.edu

Sleep Med Clin 18 (2023) 183–199
https://doi.org/10.1016/j.jsmc.2023.01.003
1556-407X/23/© 2023 Elsevier Inc. All rights reserved.

(PDSS)[5] can be quickly administered and are commonly used in the Sleep Clinic to evaluate propensity of dozing off in certain situations to both help differentiate "sleepiness" from "fatigue" and assess severity of daytime sleepiness. The Pediatric Hypersomnolence Survey (PHS) is a newly published pediatric hypersomnolence screening survey for ages 8 to 18 years freely available with 81% sensitivity and 81% specificity for narcolepsy or idiopathic hypersomnia[6] (**Fig. 1**, Supplementary Materials 1). This survey can help health-care practitioners direct referrals to sleep clinic and/or order appropriate diagnostic testing for more timely diagnoses.

Excessive daytime sleepiness is a common complaint among adolescents in particular making it difficult to tease out those with more chronic and severe complaints. In a survey of 6483 teens (13–18 years) in the United States, a staggering 41.5% reported excessive daytime sleepiness.[7] The American Academy of Sleep Medicine published sleep duration by ages: children aged 6 to

You are being asked questions about symptoms of a possible sleep problem. Think about your last week while you were in school when choosing your answers.

Check "Often" if the symptom happens 3 times or more per week. Check "Sometimes" if the symptoms happens 1–3 times per week Check "Never" if you do not have the symptom.

Check "DNK" for do not know if you are not sure if you have the symptom.

		Often (3) (> 3/week)	Sometimes (2) (1–3/week)	Never (1) (Never noted)	DNK (0) (Do not know)
1.	I fall asleep in class	☐	☐	☐	☐
2.	I miss things in class because I am sleepy	☐	☐	☐	☐
3.	My friends tell me I fall asleep easily	☐	☐	☐	☐
4.	I fall asleep in the bus/car after school	☐	☐	☐	☐
5.	I ask to go to the nurse's office or somewhere quiet to sleep during the school day	☐	☐	☐	☐
6.	I feel weak in the knees when I laugh with my friends	☐	☐	☐	☐
7.	My voice slurs when I laugh hard	☐	☐	☐	☐
8.	My body feels weak briefly when I get excited or laugh	☐	☐	☐	☐
9.	I dream when I sleep at night	☐	☐	☐	☐
10.	My dreams seem very real	☐	☐	☐	☐
11.	When I wake up, I can't move for a few minutes	☐	☐	☐	☐
12.	I write silly things when taking notes in class because I am sleepy	☐	☐	☐	☐
13.	It takes me a long time to do my homework because I am so tired	☐	☐	☐	☐
14.	Doing homework makes me tired	☐	☐	☐	☐

Fig. 1. PHS. The full PHS and instructions can be found in Supplemental Material. Score "Often" = 3 points, "Sometime" = 2 points, "Never" = 1 point. "Do not know" responses may require further clarification/explanation about symptoms queried by the provider. A Total Score greater than 24 suggests high risk for narcolepsy or idiopathic hypersomnia. The Sleepiness Subscore (Questions 1–5 and 12) greater than 8 suggests severe daytime sleepiness and is more sensitive for idiopathic hypersomnia diagnosis than the total score. (Maski K, Worhach J, Steinhart E, et al. Development and Validation of the Pediatric Hypersomnolence Survey. Neurology. 2022;98(19):e1964-e1975.)

12 years should sleep 9 to 12 hours and teens should sleep 8 to 10 hours per 24 hours on a regular basis to promote optimal health.[8] Obtaining a clear record of habitual sleep patterns from children and caregivers, including bedtime, wake time, nap times, and sleep duration over a 2-week period (including weekdays and weekends) is necessary to distinguish disorders of hypersomnolence from more common causes of sleepiness such as insufficient sleep or circadian rhythm disorders in children and adolescents. Sleep diaries or sleep logs[9] are required for this purpose but more ideally actigraphy testing (a wristwatch device that objectively identifies sleep and wake based on motion) would also be used to ensure adequate sleep is objectively present before further diagnostic testing.[1] It is important to correct insufficient sleep or circadian rhythms disorders before sleep study testing to avoid false positives for narcolepsy or idiopathic hypersomnia. For instance, Carskadan and colleagues[10] found 2 or more sleep onset rapid eye movement (REM) periods on the multiple sleep latency testing (MSLT), a criterion for narcolepsy diagnoses, in 16% of tenth grade participants with delayed circadian rhythm. Similarly, obtaining detailed descriptions of the timing, frequency, and features of naps can be helpful to differentiate between narcolepsy and idiopathic hypersomnia. For instance, a teen who sleeps 6 hours at night and takes a 2-hour nap on returning home from school is more likely to have insufficient nocturnal sleep than a teen who habitually sleeps 8 hours at night and still requires a daytime nap(s).

Narcolepsy

Clinical features

Narcolepsy type 1 and 2 are chronic neurologic disorders characterized by symptoms of excessive daytime sleepiness, sleep-related hallucinations, sleep paralysis, disrupted nocturnal sleep, and cataplexy (in narcolepsy type 1 only; **Table 1**). Children and adolescents with narcolepsy also have abnormal physiology during sleep including findings of early entry into REM sleep after sleep onset,[11–13] a lack of the typical paralysis of REM sleep (REM sleep without atonia),[14–16] and REM sleep behavior disorder.[14] Investigators report that nearly one-third of children and adolescents with narcolepsy type 1 had REM behavior disorder with complex behavior or "pantomime-like behavior" reflecting true dream enactment. Thus, atypical parasomnia behavior presenting with stereotypical gestures, dream enactment, laughing, and/or talking that occurs throughout the night may be presenting REM behavior disorder in

narcolepsy type 1 in contrast to non-rapid eye movement NREM disorders of arousals, which typically present with confused, nonpurposeful behavior in the first third of the night.

Narcolepsy type 1 can be differentiated clinically from narcolepsy type 2 by the presence of cataplexy. Cataplexy is generalized or partial loss of muscle tone, typically triggered by strong positive emotion, including laughter, surprise, or anticipation. The weakness of cataplexy may represent intrusion of REM muscle atonia into wake.[17] Generalized cataplexy, involving most of the body, seems as slumping, melting, or slouching to the floor. More commonly, cataplexy is partial, with face, neck, or limb involvement, appearing as droopy eyelids, slurred speech, or head drop.[18] Typical cataplexy features are (1) bilateral, symmetric lasting less than 2 minutes, (2) provoked by strong emotion particularly of positive nature (ie, laughter), (3) abrupt return of muscle activity after the episode, and (4) retained consciousness.[19] Children may also have "cataplexy facies," spontaneous and prolonged hypotonic attacks of the face, jaw, and eyelids associated with tongue protrusion.[20,21] Even more rarely, pediatric cataplexy can present with positive motor activity, such as phasic muscle twitches or dyskinesias; such behavior may resemble complex motor tics with repetitive mouth opening or tongue thrusting.[21–23] Additional atypical presentations of cataplexy include static tongue protrusion, ptosis, or gait instability.[21] "Status cataplecticus" is rare state of prolonged cataplexy, lasting hours, that typically occurs following abrupt withdrawal of cataplexy-suppressing medications or in the setting of insufficient sleep and has been reported in pediatric narcolepsy type 1.[14] Symptoms of daytime sleepiness typically precede or co-occur with the first episode of cataplexy. Cataplexy can occur years and even decades after onset of daytime sleepiness and notably delayed cataplexy is reportedly more common among African-American patients.[24,25] Thus, a patient could be initially diagnosed with narcolepsy type 2 and later convert to the diagnosis of narcolepsy type 1 emphasizing the importance of continually asking about the development of cataplexy in the type 2 cohort. A clinical description consistent with cataplexy should immediately raise concern for this diagnosis (**Box 1**).

Children and adolescents with both narcolepsy type 1 and type 2 describe episodic sleep paralysis, sleep-related hallucinations, and vivid dreams or dream-reality confusion. Sleep paralysis is the inability to move arms or legs for a few minutes, typically on waking from sleep, and can be present in up to 60% of people with narcolepsy.[26] People

Table 1
Clinical characteristics and diagnostic evaluation of central disorders of hypersomnolence

	Narcolepsy Type 1	Narcolepsy Type 2	Idiopathic Hypersomnia
Clinical features			
Symptom pattern	Chronic	Chronic	Chronic
Excessive daytime sleepiness	Always	Always	Always
Cataplexy	Often	Never	Never
Sleep-related hallucinations	Often	Less common	Occasional
Sleep paralysis	Often	Less common	Occasional
Disrupted nighttime sleep	Often	Less common	Rare
Prolonged sleep duration	Rare	Occasional	Often
Sleep inertia	Rare	Occasional	Often
Daytime naps	Often: brief, refreshing	Variable	Often: long, unrefreshing
Diagnostic testing			
PSG/MSLT	Sleep latency ≤8 min 2 or more SOREMPs	Sleep latency ≤8 min 2 or more SOREMPs	Sleep latency ≤ 8 min 1–1 SOREMPs Alternative: ≥11 h in 24-h PSG, or average ≥ 11 h over 1-wk actigraphy
CSF Orexin (hypocretin)	Low (<110 pg/mL)	Normal, sometimes intermediate	Normal (usually >200 pg/mL)

Abbreviations: CSF, cerebrospinal fluid; MSLT, multiple sleep latency test; PSG, polysomnography; SOREMP, sleep-onset REM period.

retain full recall of the event and are completely aware during sleep paralysis and some people may describe a sensation of someone sitting on them or preventing them from moving. As sleep paralysis can occur with sleep-related hallucinations, it can be distressing. Sleep paralysis is more common in narcolepsy type 1 than in narcolepsy type 2, and is rarer, although can be seen, in idiopathic hypersomnia.[27,28] Sleep-related hallucinations while falling asleep (hypnogogic) or waking up (hypnopompic) are similarly described in both narcolepsy types 1 and 2 and less commonly with idiopathic hypersomnia.[27,28] Hallucinations are typically visual but auditory and somatic hallucinations have also been reported by people with narcolepsy. Children and adolescents may report shadowy figures in the room, animals, or formed shapes at the time of falling asleep or waking up.[29] Sleep paralysis and sleep-related hallucinations can be described in otherwise healthy sleepers experiencing sleep deprivation and/or severe sleep disruption.[30,31] The narcolepsy "tetrad" of sleepiness, cataplexy, sleep paralysis, and sleep-related hallucinations is present in only about 45% of people with narcolepsy type 1, and all 4 features are rarely present at the same time

at the initial clinical evaluation.[28] Dream–reality confusion and vivid or lucid dreams (dreams during which a person is consciously aware of dreaming) are also reported by people with narcolepsy.[32] Occasionally, these dreams in people with narcolepsy are so realistic that they produce false memories of the dreamt events.[33] At time of symptom onset, children and adolescents with narcolepsy can have prolonged sleep duration but this normalizes with time to age-appropriate amounts of sleep.[34] Typically, children and adolescents with narcolepsy report daytime naps feel refreshing especially when naps are brief (<20 minutes).

Disrupted nocturnal sleep is a central feature of narcolepsy[35] and is enabled by intrinsic sleep instability associated with orexin (hypocretin) insufficiency.[36,37] The true prevalence of disrupted nighttime sleep in narcolepsy depends on how it is defined. Based on self-report, nearly 50% of children with narcolepsy type 1 report disrupted nighttime sleep.[38] People with narcolepsy have increased arousal index, sleep stage transitions, NREM stage 1 sleep (N1, light sleep), and wake after sleep onset time relative to healthy sleepers, subjectively sleepy controls, and people with

---

Box 1
Clinical features and causes of cataplexy in children and adolescents

Presentation of cataplexy:

Bilateral, usually symmetric weakness of face, neck, limbs

  Partial: eyelids drooping, slurred speech, head drop

  General: slouching or slumping to the floor/seated position

Atypical or positive movements:

  Dyskinetic movements or phasic muscle twitching

  Cataplexy facies

  Status cataplecticus

Decreased/absent reflexes in affected areas

Lasts seconds to minutes

Fully conscious, full event recall

Triggered by strong emotion (usually positive: laughter, anticipation)

Causes:

Strongly associated with narcolepsy type 1

Also seen in:

  Niemann-Pick type C Disease

  Angelman syndrome

  Norrie disease

  Prader-Willi syndrome

  Myotonic dystrophy

  Hypothalamic lesions: stroke, trauma, malignancy, infectious, inflammatory

---

idiopathic hypersomnia.[39–42] There is lower overall sleep efficiency in narcolepsy type 1 than either narcolepsy type 2 or idiopathic hypersomnia.[43] In particular, REM and NREM stage 2 (N2) sleep are particularly unstable in pediatric narcolepsy type 1, whereas children and adolescents with narcolepsy type 2 have more stable N1 sleep compared with subjectively sleepy controls.[41] Overall, people with narcolepsy type 2 can have clinically intermediate symptoms, with lower rates of sleep paralysis, sleep-related hallucinations, and disrupted nocturnal sleep when compared with narcolepsy type 1 (although elevated rates of these symptoms relative to healthy sleepers).[27]

Epidemiology
The prevalence of narcolepsy type 1 is estimated to be about 1:2000, or 0.05%[44] and affects men

and women equally. Age of onset is bimodal with peaks at about 15 and 35 years of age[45]; however, there is often considerable delay between symptom onset and diagnosis with median time to diagnosis as high as 10 years.[46,47] Although historically the incidence of narcolepsy type 1 was greater than narcolepsy type 2,[48,49] a recent review of the United States population showed that narcolepsy type 2 is 4.7 time more diagnosed than narcolepsy type 1 with higher reporting of women having narcolepsy type 2.[50]

Pathophysiology
Narcolepsy type 1 is caused by immune-mediated selective loss of orexin (hypocretin)-producing neurons in the hypothalamus.[51] Orexin (hypocretin) is a peptide that promotes wake and coordinates sleep-stage transition stability. In narcolepsy type 1, neuronal loss is specific to the orexin (hypocretin) neurons within the hypothalamus and even intermingling melanin-concentrating hormone neurons remain preserved.[51] Evidence supporting immune-mediated loss of these neurons includes association with specific HLA alleles (the strongest association with DQB1*0602)[52] and identification of activated T cells in people with narcolepsy type 1.[53] Additionally, there are associations of narcolepsy type 1 with T cell function identified on genome-wide association study, including components of T-cell antigen presentation and recognition.[54] Increase in narcolepsy type 1 incidence in spring (after winter virus season),[55] associations with H1N1 infection and a specific version of the H1N1 vaccine used in Europe,[56] and associations with other infectious titers further support immune-mediated cause.[52]

Narcolepsy type 2 is a clinically heterogenous disorder, and the physiology is unclear. A subset of people (about 20%) initially diagnosed with narcolepsy type 2 eventually develop orexin (hypocretin) deficiency,[57] suggesting this is an intermediate diagnosis for some. For most people with narcolepsy type 2, orexin (hypocretin) levels are normal, although there may be partial loss of orexin (hypocretin) neurons as reflected by mildly lower cerebrospinal fluid (CSF) orexin (hypocretin) levels than normal.[58]

Common comorbidities
Children and adolescents with narcolepsy often have increased risk of medical, sleep, and psychiatric comorbidities complicating disease course and treatment. Obesity is markedly high among children and adolescents with narcolepsy with prevalence of up to 74%.[59,60] In another study, additional metabolic derangements have been reported among people with narcolepsy including

increased findings of diabetes mellitus, hypertension, and dyslipidemia[61] that may increase later cardiovascular risks. Independent of obesity, investigators report precocious puberty in 17% of children and adolescents with narcolepsy.[60] Other comorbidities reported in adults with narcolepsy include thyroid dyscrasias, nonmigranous headaches, peripheral neuropathy, and chronic low back pain.[62] Sleep disorders, including obstructive sleep apnea, periodic limb movement disorder, and REM behavior disorder also have increased incidence in people with narcolepsy.[63] Psychiatric and behavioral comorbidities associated with narcolepsy include depression, anxiety, attention deficit hyperactivity disorder (ADHD), or obsessive-compulsive disorder; these conditions often persist despite treatment of daytime sleepiness.[64,65] In one study, rates of clinically significant ADHD were 15% in children and adolescents with narcolepsy type 1 and 30% in children and adolescents with narcolepsy type 2, compared with 5% to 6% of controls.[64] Given narcolepsy medication treatments can have psychiatric adverse effects, clinicians must closely monitor children and adolescents with narcolepsy for worsening or new onset mood disorders and suicidality.

Secondary narcolepsy
Cases of secondary narcolepsy or genetic conditions causing cataplexy should also be considered in the correct clinical context. Damage of the orexin (hypocretin) neurons or their projections by trauma, malignancy, inflammation, or infection can cause secondary narcolepsy with or without cataplexy in both adults and children.[66–70] Children and adolescents with cataplexy who have focal neurologic deficits or encephalopathy merit further evaluation, minimally, with brain MRI to evaluate for secondary narcolepsy. Cataplexy can be seen in neurogenetic syndromes: Niemann-Pick type C, Angelman syndrome, Norrie disease, Prader-Willi syndrome, myotonic dystrophy, and DNA methyltransferase-1 (DNMT1)-complex disorder.[71–74]

Idiopathic Hypersomnia

Clinical features
Idiopathic hypersomnia is clinically characterized by excessive daytime sleepiness, severe difficulty waking from sleep (sleep inertia), and daytime "brain fog" or cognitive cloudiness. Descriptions of the daytime sleepiness in idiopathic hypersomnia range from mild to severe and additionally, people frequently report fatigue or low energy. People with idiopathic hypersomnia can have prolonged sleep duration with more than 10 to

11 hours of habitual nocturnal sleep plus long daytime naps, yet they still report unrefreshing sleep and not feeling rested after naps[75,76] in contrast to people with narcolepsy.

Sleep inertia, or difficulty rising from sleep in the morning, is a common complaint in idiopathic hypersomnia.[77] Sleep inertia is brief in healthy sleepers[78] but in people with idiopathic hypersomnia, this period is both prolonged and pronounced. People with idiopathic hypersomnia may require multiple alarms and intervention of a family member to get them out of bed in the morning.[79] Sleep inertia in idiopathic hypersomnia is also referred to as sleep drunkenness,[80] due to cognitive dysfunction and sometimes clumsiness of movements.

Epidemiology
Idiopathic hypersomnia is thought to be a rare disease, although estimated prevalence is limited by heterogeneous symptoms; it is estimated to be about one-tenth to one-half as common as narcolepsy with 20 to 50 cases per million.[75,81–83] Symptoms often begin in the second decade, with mean onset of symptoms 19.1 years (SD 11.3 years) reported in an idiopathic hypersomnia patient registry.[84] A subset of people with idiopathic hypersomnia report symptom onset after a preceding illness or minor head trauma.[75,81] Based on a disease registry study, people with idiopathic hypersomnia tend to be female and Caucasian but demographics may be misrepresented based on survey respondents.[84]

Pathophysiology
The pathophysiology of idiopathic hypersomnia is unknown as its name implies. There are several hypotheses regarding possible mechanisms that may underlie symptoms of idiopathic hypersomnia, including enhanced gamma-aminobutyric acid (GABA) responsiveness, autonomic dysfunction, or circadian disruption. People with idiopathic hypersomnia (as well as other hypersomnia conditions) have shown increased GABA-A receptor potentiation relative to controls[85] although findings are not consistent in the literature.[86] In clinical trials, medications that modulate GABA-A receptor activity decrease sleepiness in some people with idiopathic hypersomnia.[87,88] Dysautonomia may underlie idiopathic hypersomnia physiology: people with idiopathic hypersomnia have increased autonomic symptoms relative to controls.[79,89] There is also evidence of increase in the ratio of parasympathetic to sympathetic activity in idiopathic hypersomnia in a study of heart rate variability.[90] Another hypothesis is that idiopathic hypersomnia represents a circadian rhythm disorder, with data supporting a "long biologic night."

Skin fibroblasts from people with idiopathic hypersomnia have prolonged circadian period length relative to controls[91] and decreased amplitude of circadian gene expression.[92] A challenge in identifying the cause of idiopathic hypersomnia may be the heterogeneity in the patient population but possibly there are diverse pathophysiology and mechanisms resulting in a common phenotype.

There is ongoing discussion regarding the relationship between narcolepsy type 2 and idiopathic hypersomnia, and a subset of these people (especially those with normal sleep duration) may share common physiology.[93] Currently diagnostic differentiation between these conditions is reliant on the presence of 2 or more sleep onset REM periods (SOREMPs) on the polysomnogram (PSG) and MSLT (detailed further below) for narcolepsy. However, the MSLT test-retest reliability can be poor in adults with idiopathic hypersomnia and narcolepsy type 2[94–96] and therefore difficulties differentiating these conditions may be due to testing limitations. It is unknown if similar MSLT reliability issues are present in pediatric patient populations.

DIAGNOSTIC TOOLS AND EVALUATION FOR NARCOLEPSY AND IDIOPATHIC HYPERSOMNIA

In addition to the sleep history, disorders of hypersomnolence are most commonly diagnosed by overnight PSG followed by the MSLT. The overnight PSG helps to exclude factors that contribute to daytime sleepiness, such as sleep apnea or sleep deprivation (a minimum of 6 hours of sleep is required on overnight PSG to proceed with the MSLT), and to record REM sleep latency because this may be used toward the diagnosis of narcolepsy. The MSLT consists of five 20-minute nap opportunities every 2 hours throughout the day (**Fig. 2**) and measures sleep latency and SOREMPs. A mean sleep onset latency consistent with hypersomnolence is defined as less than or equal to 8 minutes in both narcolepsy and idiopathic hypersomnia. A sleep onset REM period is defined as the onset of REM sleep occurring within 15 minutes of falling asleep (SOREMP). Narcolepsy is distinguished from idiopathic hypersomnia by the presence of 2 or more SOREMPs in either the nap opportunities of the MSLT or the beginning of the overnight PSG (nocturnal SOREMP). In a study of children and adolescents undergoing evaluation for suspected narcolepsy, at least 2 SOREMPs *or* a mean sleep latency less than or equal to 8.2 minutes on the MSLT were reliable markers for pediatric narcolepsy type 1.[97] The nocturnal SOREMP is an important biomarker for

adults and children with narcolepsy with cataplexy with high specificity (97%) but relatively poor sensitivity less than 60%.[11,13] The high specificity of this nocturnal SOREMP biomarker permits diagnosis of narcolepsy with only PSG alone in the Diagnostic and Statistical Manual of Mental Disorders, Fifth Edition.[98]

Several scenarios can result in a false-positive PSG-MSLT testing. In particular, habitual sleep timings (weekdays and weekends) and duration can influence results as noted in the "Initial Approach to the Sleepy Child/Adolescent" section. Actigraphy or sleep logs should be obtained for the 2 weeks leading up to the sleep study.[99] Further, medications impact sleep architecture and can influence the MSLT. Medications that are sedating or alerting can impact sleep onset latency. SOREMPs can also be influenced by medications, most commonly selective serotonin reuptake inhibitors (SSRI) antidepressants, which suppress REM sleep.[100,101] In a pediatric study of MSLT outcomes, patients on REM-suppressing antidepressants had fewer SOREMPs than those not taking these medications.[102] Of note, withdrawal effects of REM-suppressing antidepressants with an advanced taper can influence the MSLT by increasing the numbers of MSLT SOREMPs and reducing mean sleep latency.[102] Tapering REM-suppressing medications are less important for the evaluation of idiopathic hypersomnia because REM abnormalities are not part of the diagnostic criteria. Optimally, any medications that impact sleep propensity and sleep architecture should be tapered before testing; whereas 2-weeks is recommended for most antidepressants,[103] and this may not be sufficient for medications with longer half-lives such as fluoxetine. Illicit drug use and withdrawal as well as caffeine use can also influence sleep latency and REM sleep,[104,105] so urine toxicology screening is routinely obtained on the morning of the MSLT.

To address these many contextual influencers, the American Academy of Sleep Medicine developed updated 2021 practice parameters to guide testing.[99] These include guidelines for the study night, as well as preparation. Specifically, the guidelines recommend a 2-week activity/sleep log (and actigraphy when able) and 2-week tapering off of REM suppressing/sleep altering medications. These guidelines also recommend the MSLT report author detail medication used or recently discontinued on the MSLT report to improve transparency of potentially confounding factors for clinical interpretation.[99] Overall, the MSLT has high diagnostic validity and reliability for people with narcolepsy type 1[95]; however, there is more variability for diagnosis of narcolepsy

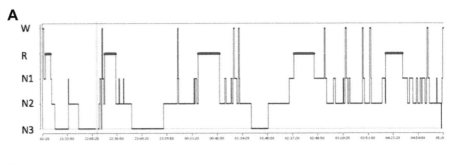

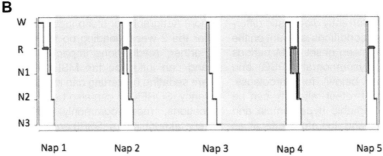

Fig. 2. Overnight PSG and MSLT of a patient with narcolepsy. (*A*) Overnight PSG shows a nocturnal sleep onset REM period (defined by REM sleep within 15 minutes of sleep onset, which is a biomarker for narcolepsy. Sensitivity is 55% and specificity is 97% in children aged 6–18 years with narcolepsy type 1 (Andlauer 2013, Reiter 2015). (*B*) MSLT includes a series of five 20-minute nap opportunities at 2-hour intervals.

type 2 and idiopathic hypersomnia.[34,106] For people with idiopathic hypersomnia, the sensitivity of the MSLT is low, and the test-re-test reliability is similarly poor.[94–96] For these individuals, alternative diagnostic testing or new biomarkers are needed.

Within the ICSD3, diagnosis of idiopathic hypersomnia is also possible with documentation of prolonged sleep duration on either extended PSG or actigraphy as an acceptable alternative to the MSLT criteria. Extended sleep duration is defined as 11 hours on both extended PSG (up to 24 hours) or as averaged over 7 days on actigraphy. There is data to suggest that long sleep time measured on extended PSG has superior sensitivity in idiopathic hypersomnia.[107] These 24 to 36-hour protocols provide improved diagnostic accuracy and reliability; however, they are rarely feasible in clinical sleep laboratories, not currently reimbursed, and not validated for pediatric idiopathic hypersomnia. Actigraphy uses motion to estimate sleep–wake patterns and has been studied in central disorders of hypersomnolence,[108,109] and although it has the advantage of measuring sleep wake in the home setting, it is not widely available due to cost and limited reimbursement. Of note, this diagnostic pathway is based only on clinical actigraphs, not direct-to-consumer devices,[110] and has not been validated in children or adolescents.

Alternative Evaluation

In addition to neurophysiologic testing, for a select group of people with hypersomnolence and suspicion for narcolepsy type 1, CSF testing for orexin (hypocretin) level may be diagnostic. In children and adolescents with daytime sleepiness, low CSF orexin (hypocretin) level (<110 pg/mL) alone is sufficient for the diagnosis of narcolepsy type 1.[57] For example, CSF orexin (hypocretin) testing may be a useful alternative diagnostic pathway for a patient with clinical episodes consistent with cataplexy who is unable to undergo the MSLT, or unable to taper off of REM-altering medications in preparation for the MSLT. Orexin (hypocretin) levels are (by definition) greater than 110 pg/mL in narcolepsy type 2; if a patient with suspected narcolepsy type 2 has CSF testing with low orexin (hypocretin), the diagnosis changes to narcolepsy type 1. In children, sleepiness often precedes cataplexy, and the presence of low CSF orexin alone would be diagnostic for narcolepsy type 1; these children and adolescents can be counseled that they may develop cataplexy over time.

Serum human leukocyte antigen (HLA) testing can have some clinical utility. Narcolepsy type 1 has a strong association with HLA-DQ1B*06:02, which is present in 98% of people with narcolepsy type 1,[57,111] although this is also seen in up to 30%

of healthy sleepers[111] and is most useful when negative to exclude diagnosis. Because it is rare to see narcolepsy type 1 without this HLA positivity, CSF orexin (hypocretin) is very unlikely to be low and lumbar puncture would be of low yield. HLA-DQ1B*06:02 may be either present in 40% to 60% of people with narcolepsy type 2.[112,113]

Clinical scales have been validated for use in the assessment of symptom frequency, severity, and burden for pediatric narcolepsy (The Pediatric Narcolepsy Severity Scale[114] validated in children aged 10 years and older) and for idiopathic hypersomnia (the Idiopathic Hypersomnia Severity Scale[115] validated in adolescents and adults aged 16 years and older). Of note, these scales query symptoms beyond severity of daytime sleepiness, such as cataplexy, sleep paralysis, and sleep-related hallucinations in narcolepsy, and sleep inertia and daytime naps in idiopathic hypersomnia. Both of these severity scales show treatment sensitivity. Otherwise, other commonly used validated instruments for excessive daytime sleepiness used for pediatric outcome measurement include the ESS-CHAD[4] (Janssen 2017) and the PDSS.[5]

Disease Management

There are currently no cures for narcolepsy or idiopathic hypersomnia, and the therapeutic goals are to improve sleepiness and other burdensome symptoms to optimize academic/work, social, and familial functioning. For daytime sleepiness, there are both pharmacologic and behavioral approaches to lessen symptom severity. Medications selection should be individualized to the patient's risk/benefit ratio, cost, and potential adverse effects with existing comorbidities. Nonpharmacologic interventions including maintaining a regular sleep schedule, avoiding sedating daytime medications/substances, lifestyle adjustments, physical activity, and inclusion of academic accommodations are important for all children and adolescents with hypersomnolence. Scheduled daytime naps, 15 to 30 minutes duration, can temporarily improve excessive daytime sleepiness and improve alertness in children and adolescents with narcolepsy. Naps are typically less helpful for sleepiness mitigation in idiopathic hypersomnia because of difficulty waking from naps and sleep inertia. **Box 2** includes sample school accommodations for children and adolescents with narcolepsy and idiopathic hypersomnia.

Treatment of Pediatric Narcolepsy

For children and adolescents with narcolepsy, the only United States Food and Drug Administration

---

Box 2
Helpful accommodations for children and adolescents with narcolepsy or idiopathic hypersomnia

Children

1. Consider a study period during the academic day. This allows patients to get more work done while medications are active and permits time for naps as needed.

2. Have patient sit at front of class to help with vigilance. Alternatively, some children prefer sitting in back of classroom so they can take a scheduled nap.

3. Schedule a 30-minute nap during the day in quiet, safe area in school. Patients typically benefit from this nap after lunch or early afternoon.

4. Allow patients to chew gum, drink cool water, and/or take movement breaks during class/test taking to maintain alertness.

5. Request extra time for completion of homework/tests/projects. Patients need to keep 9 to 10 hours for sleep at night and this can be difficult if they are overwhelmed by homework responsibility.

6. Maintain exercise daily as exercise.

Adolescents/College Students

1. Priority registration for high school/college courses so patients can schedule classes for when they are most alert.

2. Provision of class notes/audio recordings if patient is too sleepy to pay attention in class.

3. Private dorm room for undisturbed sleep at night.

4. A dorm room close to classes so patients can take scheduled naps.

(FDA) approved therapies are traditional stimulant medications (amphetamines, methylphenidate) for treatment of daytime sleepiness and sodium oxybate or lower sodium oxybate (calcium, magnesium, potassium, and sodium oxybates) for the treatment of excessive daytime sleepiness and cataplexy (7–17 years). Based on a meta-analysis of available pediatric clinical trials, the American Academy of Sleep Medicine issued clinical practice guidelines for the treatment of pediatric narcolepsy.[116] These guidelines issued conditional recommendations for the use of modafinil for the treatment of daytime sleepiness and sodium oxybate for the treatment of excessive daytime sleepiness and cataplexy. The lack of clinical trials with sufficient number of participants and/or use of validated instruments limited the

Table 2
Treatments of narcolepsy and idiopathic hypersomnia in children and adolescents (excessive daytime sleepiness and cataplexy

Medication	Dose	Side Effects
Stimulants		
Methylphenidate immediate release	10–60 mg/d in 2–3 divided doses	Common: anorexia, poor growth or weight loss, sleep disturbance, jitteriness, tics, emotional lability
Methylphenidate ER or SR	20–60 mg/d	
Methylphenidate (concerta)	18–54 mg/d	
Methylphenidate (patch)	10–30 mg/d	Rare, serious: psychosis, mania, seizure, priapism, cardiovascular effects
Dextroamphetamine IR	5–40 mg/d in 1–2 divided doses	
Amphetamine/ dextroamphetamine IR	10–40 mg/d in 1–2 divided doses	Monitor blood pressure, caution if family or personal history of cardiac arrhythmias
Lisdexamfetamine	30–70 mg/d	
Wake-promoting medications		
Modafinil	50–200 mg in 1–2 divided doses	Common: headache, nervousness, nausea, insomnia
Armodafinil	50–250 mg in 1–2 divided doses	Rare, serious: severe rash (Stevens-Johnson syndrome), psychiatric events
		CYP3A4/5 induction: impair effectiveness of steroidal contraceptives
		Exposure during pregnancy increases risk of congenital malformations
Others		
Sodium oxybate, lower-sodium oxybate	2–9 g/night in 2 divided doses 20–30 kg: 6 g max 30–45 kg: 7.5 g max >45 kg: 9 g max	Common: morning sedation, nausea, weight loss, dizziness, enuresis, sleep walking, tremor, constipation, worsening of obstructive sleep apnea (OSA)
		Rare, serious: confusion, severe sedation, coma
		Not to be used with alcohol, sedatives, or hypnotics
		Central pharmacy with enrollment in REMS program
Atomoxetine	0.5–1.2 mg/kg/d in 1–2 divided doses (max, 100 mg/d)	Common: weight loss, abdominal pain, nausea, anorexia, headache
		Rare, serious: suicidal ideation, psychosis, mania, cardiovascular events, priapism, hepatotoxicity
Medication	**Dose[a]**	**Side Effects**
Sodium oxybate, lower-sodium oxybate	2–9 g/night in 2 divided doses 20–30 kg: 6 g max 30–45 kg: 7.5 g max >45 kg: 9 g max	Common: morning sedation, nausea, weight loss, dizziness, enuresis, sleep walking, tremor, constipation, worsening of OSA
		Rare, serious: confusion, severe sedation, coma
		Not to be used with alcohol, sedatives, or hypnotics

(continued on next page)

Table 2
(*continued*)

Medication	Dose[a]	Side Effects

Tricyclic antidepressants
  Clomipramine
  Imipramine
  Protriptyline
	25–100 mg/d at bedtime
	25–75 mg/d, 2 divided doses
	5–10 mg/d in 1–2 divided doses
		Common: dry mouth, constipation, diaphoresis, blurred vision, somnolence, weight gain, orthostatic hypotension
		Rare, serious: cardiotoxicity, suicidal ideation, bone marrow suppression, serotonin syndrome

Selective serotonin reuptake inhibitors
  Fluoxetine
  Sertraline
  Citalopram
	10–30 mg/d
	25–200 mg/d
	10–40 mg/d
		Common: nausea, insomnia, tremor
		Rare, serious: suicidal ideation, QT prolongation, serotonin syndrome

Serotonin norepinephrine reuptake inhibitors Venlafaxine	37.5–75 mg/d	Common: nausea, weight loss, dizziness, headache, constipation, insomnia, somnolence, tremor Rare, serious: suicidal ideation, QT prolongation, serotonin syndrome

[a] Doses for children aged 6 years and older, except clomipramine and protriptyline, which are for ages 10 and older.

ability to include recommendations for traditional stimulants and daytime naps for excessive daytime sleepiness treatment and SSRI/SNRI commonly used for cataplexy control. In clinical practice, stimulants are often the first-line therapy, based on US FDA approval. There are no longitudinal data regarding stimulant use in pediatric narcolepsy but clinical experience suggests children and adolescents can have short-term side effects including delayed sleep onset, reduced appetite, headaches, weight loss, and potential for worsening of comorbid conditions such as anxiety and depression. Long-term use seems safe in children with primary attention hyperactivity disorder with close follow-up but data have been inconsistent regarding the potential of stimulant growth effects.[117] Modafinil or armodafinil for excessive daytime sleepiness is typically second-line therapy if there is inadequate response or intolerance to stimulants. Although modafinil and armodafinil are not FDA-approved for patients under 18 years due to concerns of Stevens Johnson syndrome and psychosis, observational studies suggest significant symptomatic improvement of daytime sleepiness in pediatric narcolepsy and only minor side effects.[118–120] Use of sodium oxybate for pediatric narcolepsy has been the only medication studied in a randomized, placebo-controlled, clinical trial study,[121] and the study showed significant improvements in excessive daytime sleepiness

and cataplexy from baseline with sodium oxybate use. There were rare adverse serious effects in this clinical trial including central sleep apnea, depression, and suicidality; more common side effects are listed in **Table 2**. Clinicians are required to enroll in a Risk Evaluation and Mitigation Strategies (REMS) program before receiving sodium oxybate. Lower-sodium oxybate was FDA-approved in 2020 for children aged 7 years and older and can be used with similar efficacy and tolerability as sodium oxybate. Lower-sodium oxybate could be considered if there is a concern about the high sodium content of sodium oxybate (about 1640 mg/d compared with 131 mg sodium at the maximal dose, 9 mg), such in cases of patients with elevated blood pressure or risk factors for hypertension.

Overall, given reports of increased cardiovascular disease in adults with narcolepsy,[122] close monitoring of blood pressure is recommended with narcolepsy treatments discussed. Newer treatments approved for adults with narcolepsy include solriamfetol and pitolisant. Pitolisant is a selective histamine 3 receptor antagonist/inverse agonist, and decreases cataplexy and sleepiness in adults,[123] although it is not yet been approved for children pending clinical trial data. A small case series suggests safety and improvement of daytime sleepiness and in children with Prader-Willi syndrome.[124] Solriamfetol, a selective dopamine and norepinephrine reuptake inhibitor also improves sleepiness in adults with narcolepsy but has not been studied in children.[125,126] Orexin agonists are currently in clinical trial phases and may offer more effective therapies in the future.[127]

Commonly used medications for symptoms of daytime sleepiness and cataplexy, dosages, and associated side effects are summarized in **Table 2**.

Treatment of Pediatric Idiopathic Hypersomnia

There are no pharmacologic treatment options studied for pediatric idiopathic hypersomnia and no FDA-approved therapies. In adults, lower-sodium oxybate was recently approved for treatment of idiopathic hypersomnia based on a multicenter study of 154 adults aged 18-75 years (median age 39 years) showing improvement of excessive daytime sleepiness on the Epworth Sleepiness Score from the end of the stable dose period to the end of the double-blind, randomized, withdrawal period.[128] Additionally, lower-sodium oxybate was associated with benefits to overall idiopathic hypersomnia symptoms and patient impression of symptom severity relative to the placebo control.[128] The American Academy of Sleep Medicine clinical practice guidelines for the treatment of central disorders of hypersomnolence (published before this oxybate study) includes a recommendation for modafinil for the treatment of idiopathic hypersomnia in adults based on 1 randomized control trial and 3 observational studies.[116] There are less data to support the use of methylphenidate, pitolisant, or clarithromycin in adults with idiopathic hypersomnia.[116]

In clinical practice, clinicians typically treat the excessive daytime sleepiness in pediatric idiopathic hypersomnia with stimulants, modafinil, or armodafinil using similar guidance detailed in the narcolepsy section above. Similar accommodations as listed in **Box 2** can be applied for children and adolescents with idiopathic hypersomnia. Certainly, more study and clinical trial data are needed to guide pediatric practitioners in optimal pediatric idiopathic hypersomnia management.

SUMMARY

Narcolepsy and idiopathic hypersomnia have significant impact on optimal participation in school and social and family interactions. Obtaining a detailed clinical sleep history from children and adolescents and their caregivers is critical for early recognition of these disorders. Thoughtful interpretation of neurophysiologic testing is needed for accurate diagnosis of narcolepsy and idiopathic hypersomnia. Tailoring treatment approaches to meet the needs of individuals and account for medical and psychiatric comorbidities may also improve quality of life.

CLINICS CARE POINTS

- Narcolepsy is a lifelong disease that often presents in adolescence or childhood results in severe daytime sleepiness that impairs physical and mental health with impact on social, academic, and professional life.

- Daytime sleepiness in children may manifest as hyperactivity, irritability, or emotional lability.

- Children and adolescents with narcolepsy may experience symptoms of REM sleep intrusion into wake, such as sleep-related hallucinations, sleep paralysis, and cataplexy.

- Cataplexy is sudden loss of muscle tone triggered by strong, usually positive, emotion. In children, cataplexy presentation may be complex or atypical with dyskinesias or motor activity.

- Narcolepsy and idiopathic hypersomnia are often diagnosed with overnight PSG followed by MSLT. Insufficient sleep, circadian rhythm disorders, and certain medications may result is false-positive testing, and this study should be interpreted in the clinical context.

- Treatment of daytime sleepiness in narcolepsy or idiopathic hypersomnia may include sleep hygiene and scheduled naps but most people require pharmacotherapy. First-line treatments for sleepiness typically include stimulants, followed by modafinil/armodafinil. If both cataplexy and sleepiness are bothersome, sodium oxybate or lower-sodium oxybate may be first-line therapy.

- Mood should be monitored closely during treatment with medications that reduce cataplexy because there may be increased suicidal ideation with the initiation of antidepressants or oxybates.

DECLARATION OF INTERESTS

M. Blattner has no relevant disclosures. K. Maski receives research support from Jazz Pharmaceuticals, Ireland and Harmony Biosciences, United States, has consulted for Jazz Pharmaceuticals, Harmony Biosciences, Takeda, KemPharm, Alkermes, and serves on the DSMB for Idorsia Pharmaceuticals.

SUPPLEMENTARY DATA

Supplementary data related to this article can be found online at https://doi.org/10.1016/j.jsmc.2023.01.003.

REFERENCES

1. International classification of sleep disorders - third edition (ICSD-3). Darien (IL): American Academy of Sleep Medicine; 2014.
2. Givan DC. The sleepy child. Pediatr Clin North Am 2004;51(1):15–31.
3. Owens JA, Babcock D, Weiss M. Evaluation and treatment of children and adolescents with excessive daytime sleepiness. Clin Pediatr 2020;59(4–5):340–51.
4. Janssen KC, Phillipson S, O'Connor J, et al. Validation of the epworth sleepiness scale for children and adolescents using rasch analysis. Sleep Med 2017;33:30–5.
5. Drake C, Nickel C, Burduvali E, et al. The pediatric daytime sleepiness scale (PDSS): sleep habits and school outcomes in middle-school children. Sleep 2003;26(4):455–8.
6. Maski K, Worhach J, Steinhart E, et al. Development and validation of the pediatric hypersomnolence survey. Neurology 2022;98(19):e1964–75.
7. Kolla BP, He J-P, Mansukhani MP, et al. Prevalence and correlates of hypersomnolence symptoms in US teens. J Am Acad Child Adolesc Psychiatry 2019;58(7):712–20.
8. Paruthi S, Brooks LJ, D'Ambrosio C, et al. Recommended amount of sleep for pediatric populations: a consensus statement of the american academy of sleep medicine. J Clin Sleep Med 2016;12(6):785–6.
9. American academy of sleep medicine: sleep education. Sleep diary. Available at: https://sleepeducation.org/resources/sleep-diary/. Accessed June 7, 2022.
10. Carskadon MA, Wolfson AR, Acebo C, et al. Adolescent sleep patterns, circadian timing, and sleepiness at a transition to early school days. Sleep 1998;21(8):871–81.
11. Andlauer O, Moore H, Jouhier L, et al. Nocturnal rapid eye movement sleep latency for identifying patients with narcolepsy/hypocretin deficiency. JAMA Neurol 2013;70(7):891–902.
12. Ferri R, Franceschini C, Zucconi M, et al. Searching for a marker of REM sleep behavior disorder: submentalis muscle EMG amplitude analysis during sleep in patients with narcolepsy/cataplexy. Sleep 2008;31(10):1409–17.
13. Reiter J, Katz E, Scammell TE, et al. Usefulness of a nocturnal SOREMP for diagnosing narcolepsy with cataplexy in a pediatric population. Sleep 2015;38(6):859–65.
14. Antelmi E, Pizza F, Vandi S, et al. The spectrum of REM sleep-related episodes in children with type 1 narcolepsy. Brain 2017;140(6):1669–79.
15. Bin-Hasan S, Videnovic A, Maski K. Nocturnal REM sleep without atonia is a diagnostic biomarker of pediatric narcolepsy. J Clin Sleep Med 2018;14(2):245–52.
16. Dauvilliers Y, Jennum P, Plazzi G. Rapid eye movement sleep behavior disorder and rapid eye movement sleep without atonia in narcolepsy. Sleep Med 2013;14(8):775–81.
17. Dauvilliers Y, Siegel JM, Lopez R, et al. Cataplexy–clinical aspects, pathophysiology and management strategy. Nat Rev Neurol 2014;10(7):386–95.
18. Overeem S, SJv Nues, Zande WLvd, et al. The clinical features of cataplexy: a questionnaire study in narcolepsy patients with and without hypocretin-1 deficiency. Sleep Med 2011;12(1):12–8.
19. van der Hoeven AE, Fronczek R, Schinkelshoek MS, et al. Intermediate hypocretin-1 cerebrospinal fluid levels and typical cataplexy: their significance in the diagnosis of narcolepsy type 1. Sleep 2022;45(5):zsac052.
20. Prasad M, Setty G, Ponnusamy A, et al. Cataplectic facies: clinical marker in the diagnosis of childhood narcolepsy-report of two cases. Pediatr Neurol 2014;50(5):515–7.
21. Serra L, Montagna P, Mignot E, et al. Cataplexy features in childhood narcolepsy. Mov Disord 2008;23(6):858–65.
22. Kryger MH, Walid R, Manfreda J. Diagnoses received by narcolepsy patients in the year prior to diagnosis by a sleep specialist. Sleep 2002;25(1):36–41.
23. Plazzi G, Pizza F, Palai V, et al. Complex movement disorders at disease onset in childhood narcolepsy with cataplexy. Brain 2011;134:3477–89.
24. Andlauer O, 4th HM, Hong S-C, et al. Predictors of hypocretin (orexin) deficiency in narcolepsy without cataplexy. Sleep 2012;35(9):1247–55.
25. Kawai M, O'Hara R, Einen M, et al. Narcolepsy in African Americans. Sleep 2015;38(11):1673–81.
26. Kim LJ, Coelho FM, Hirotsu C, et al. Frequencies and associations of narcolepsy-related symptoms: a cross-sectional study. J Clin Sleep Med 2015;11(12):1377–84.
27. Khan Z, Trotti LM. Central disorders of hypersomnolence: focus on the narcolepsies and idiopathic hypersomnia. Chest 2015;148(1):262–73.
28. Luca G, Haba-Rubio J, Dauvilliers Y, et al. Clinical, polysomnographic and genome-wide association analyses of narcolepsy with cataplexy: a European Narcolepsy Network study. J Sleep Res 2013;22(5):482–95.
29. Plazzi G, Fabbri C, Pizza F, et al. Schizophrenia-like symptoms in narcolepsy type 1: shared and distinctive

clinical characteristics. Neuropsychobiology 2015; 71(4):218–24.

30. Denis D, French CC, Gregory AM. A systematic review of variables associated with sleep paralysis. Sleep Med Rev 2018;38:141–57.

31. Sharpless BA, Barberb JP. Lifetime prevalence rates of sleep paralysis: a systematic review. Sleep Med Rev 2011;15(5):311–5.

32. Dodet P, Chavez M, Leu-Semenescu S, et al. Lucid dreaming in narcolepsy. Sleep 2015;38(3): 487–97.

33. Wamsley E, Donjacour CEHM, Scammell TE, et al. Delusional confusion of dreaming and reality in narcolepsy. Sleep 2014;37(2):419–22.

34. Pizza F, Franceschini C, Peltola H, et al. Clinical and polysomnographic course of childhood narcolepsy with cataplexy. Brain 2013;136:3787–95.

35. Maski K, Mignot E, Plazzi G, et al. Disrupted nighttime sleep and sleep instability in narcolepsy. J Clin Sleep Med 2022;18(1):289–304.

36. Barateau L, Lopez R, Chenini S, et al. Association of CSF orexin-A levels and nocturnal sleep stability in patients with hypersomnolence. Neurology 2020; 95(21):e2900–11.

37. Behn CGD, Klerman EB, Mochizuki T, et al. Abnormal sleep/wake dynamics in orexin knockout mice. Sleep 2010;33(3):297–306.

38. Pizza F, Peltola H, Sarkanen T, et al. Childhood narcolepsy with cataplexy: comparison between post-H1N1 vaccination and sporadic cases. Sleep Med 2014;15(2):262–5.

39. Bruck D, Parkes JD. A comparison of idiopathic hypersomnia and narcolepsy-cataplexy using self report measures and sleep diary data. J Neurol Neurosurg Psychiatr 1996;60(5):576–8.

40. Maski K., Pizza F., Liu S., et al., Defining disrupted nighttime sleep and assessing its diagnostic utility for pediatric narcolepsy type 1, *Sleep*, 43 (10), 2020, 1-7.

41. Maski KP, Colclasure A, Little E, et al. Stability of nocturnal wake and sleep stages defines central nervous system disorders of hypersomnolence. Sleep 2021;44(7).

42. Roth T, Dauvilliers Y, Mignot E, et al. Disrupted nighttime sleep in narcolepsy. J Clin Sleep Med 2013;9(9):955–65.

43. Takei Y, Komada Y, Namba K, et al. Differences in findings of nocturnal polysomnography and multiple sleep latency test between narcolepsy and idiopathic hypersomnia. Clin Neurophysiol 2012; 123(1):137–41.

44. Mignot E. Genetic and familial aspects of narcolepsy. Neurology 1998;50:S16–22.

45. Dauvilliers Y, Montplaisir J, Molinari N, et al. Age at onset of narcolepsy in two large populations of patients in France and Quebec. Neurology 2001; 57(11):2029–33.

46. Maski K, Steinhart E, Williams D, et al. Listening to the patient voice in narcolepsy: diagnostic delay, disease burden, and treatment efficacy. J Clin Sleep Med 2017;13(3):419–25.

47. Thorpy MJ, Krieger AC. Delayed diagnosis of narcolepsy: characterization and impact. Sleep Med 2014;15(5):502–7.

48. Silber MH, Krahn LE, Olson EJ, et al. The epidemiology of narcolepsy in olmsted county, Minnesota: a population-based study. Sleep 2002;25(2): 197–202.

49. Longstreth W, Ton TGN, Koepsell T, et al. Prevalence of narcolepsy in king count, Washington, USA. Sleep Med 2009;10(4):422–6.

50. Scheer D, Schwartz SW, Parr M, et al. Prevalence and incidence of narcolepsy in a US health care claims database, 2008-2010. Sleep 2019;42(7).

51. Thannickal TC, Moore RY, Nienhuis R, et al. Reduced number of hypocretin neurons in human narcolepsy. Neuron 2000;27(3):469–74.

52. Bassetti CLA, Adamantidis A, Burdakov D, et al. Narcolepsy - clinical spectrum, aetiopathophysiology, diagnosis and treatment. Nat Rev Neurol 2019;15(9):519–39.

53. Latorre D, Kallweit U, Armentani E, et al. T cells in patients with narcolepsy target self-antigens of hypocretin neurons. Nature 2018;562(7725):63–8.

54. Hallmayer J, Faraco J, Lin L, et al. Narcolepsy is strongly associated with the T-cell receptor alpha locus. Nat Genet 2009;41(6):708–11.

55. Wu H, Zhuang J, Stone WS, et al. Symptoms and occurrences of narcolepsy: a retrospective study of 162 patients during a 10-year period in eastern China. Sleep Med 2014;15(6):607–13.

56. Ahmed SS, Schur PH, MacDonald NE, et al. Narcolepsy, 2009 A(H1N1) pandemic influenza, and pandemic influenza vaccinations: what is known and unknown about the neurological disorder, the role for autoimmunity, and vaccine adjuvants. Journal Autoimmunology 2014;(50):1–11.

57. Han F, Lin L, Schormair B, et al. HLA DQB1*06:02 negative narcolepsy with hypocretin/orexin deficiency. Sleep 2014;37(10):1601–8.

58. Thannickal TC, Nienhuis R, Siegel JM. Localized loss of hypocretin (orexin) cells in narcolepsy without cataplexy. Sleep 2009;32(8):993–8.

59. Kotagal S, Krahn LE, Slocumb N. A putative link between childhood narcolepsy and obesity. Sleep Med 2004;5(2):147–50.

60. Poli F, Pizza F, Mignot E, et al. High prevalence of precocious puberty and obesity in childhood narcolepsy with cataplexy. Sleep 2013;36(2): 175–81.

61. Mohammadi S, Moosaie F, Saghazadeh A, et al. Metabolic profile in patients with narcolepsy: a systematic review and meta-analysis. Sleep Med 2021;81:268–84.

62. Cohen A, Mandrekar J, Louis EKS, et al. Comorbidities in a community sample of narcolepsy. Sleep Med 2018;43:14–8.

63. Sasai-Sakuma T, Kinoshita A, Inoue Y. Polysomnographic assessment of sleep comorbidities in drug-naïve narcolepsy-spectrum disorders–a Japanese cross-sectional study. PLoS One 2015; 10(8):e0136988.

64. Lecendreux M, Lavault S, Lopez R, et al. Attention-deficit/hyperactivity disorder (ADHD) symptoms in pediatric narcolepsy: a cross-sectional study. Sleep 2015;83(8):1285–95.

65. Ohayon MM. Narcolepsy is complicated by high medical and psychiatric comorbidities: a comparison with the general population. Sleep Med 2013; 14(6):488–92.

66. Compta Y, Iranzo A, Santamaría J, et al. REM sleep behavior disorder and narcoleptic features in Anti–Ma2-associated encephalitis. Sleep 2007;30(6): 767–9.

67. Dalmau J, Graus F, Villarejo A, et al. Clinical analysis of anti-Ma2-associated encephalitis. Brain 2004;127:1831–44.

68. Madan R, Pitts J, Patterson MC, et al. Secondary narcolepsy in children. J Child Neurol 2021;36(2):123–7.

69. Nishino S, Kanbayashi T. Symptomatic narcolepsy, cataplexy and hypersomnia, and their implications in the hypothalamic hypocretin/orexin system. Sleep Med Rev 2005;9(4):269–310.

70. Rosen GM, Bendel AE, Neglia JP, et al. Sleep in children with neoplasms of the central nervous system: case review of 14 children. Pediatrics 2003; 112:e46–54.

71. Bi H, Hojo K, Watanabe M, et al. Expanded genetic insight and clinical experience of DNMT1-complex disorder. Neurology Genetics 2020;6(4):e456.

72. Lima FCB Jr, do Nascimento EB Jr, Teixeira SS, et al. Thinking outside the box: cataplexy without narcolepsy. Sleep Med 2019;61:118–21.

73. Malik S, Boeve BF, Krahn LE, et al. Narcolepsy associated with other central nervous system disorders. Neurology 2001;57(3):539–41.

74. Manni R, Politini L, Nobili L, et al. Hypersomnia in the Prader Willi syndrome: clinical-electrophysiological features and underlying factors. Clin Neurophysiol 2001;112(5):800–5.

75. Anderson KN, Pilsworth S, Sharples LD, et al. Idiopathic hypersomnia: a study of 77 cases. Sleep 2007;30(10):1274–81.

76. Vernet C, Arnulf I. Idiopathic hypersomnia with and without long sleep time: a controlled series of 75 patients. Sleep 2009;32(6):753–9.

77. Trotti LM. Waking up is the hardest thing I do all day: sleep inertia and sleep drunkenness. Sleep Med Rev 2017;35:76–84.

78. Tassi P, Muzet A. Sleep inertia. Sleep Med Rev 2000;4(4):341–53.

79. Vernet C, Leu-Semenescu S, Buzare M-A, et al. Subjective symptoms in idiopathic hypersomnia: beyond excessive sleepiness. J Sleep Res 2010; 19(4):525–34.

80. Roth B, Nevsimalova S, Rechtschaffen A. Hypersomnia with "sleep drunkenness. Arch Gen Psychiatr 1972;26(5):456–62.

81. Bassetti C, Aldrich MS. Idiopathic hypersomnia. A series of 42 patients. Brain 1997;120:1423–35.

82. Billiard M. Idiopathic hypersomnia. Neurol Clin 1996;14(3):573–82.

83. Coleman RM, Roffwarg HP, Kennedy SJ, et al. Sleep-wake disorders based on a polysomnographic diagnosis. A national cooperative study. JAMA 1982;247(7):997–1003.

84. Trotti LM, Ong JC, Plante DT, et al. Disease symptomatology and response to treatment in people with idiopathic hypersomnia: initial data from the Hypersomnia Foundation registry. Sleep Med 2020;75:343–9.

85. Rye DB, Bliwise DL, Parker K, et al. Modulation of vigilance in the primary hypersomnias by endogenous enhancement of GABAA receptors. Sci Transl Med 2012;4(161):151.

86. Dauvilliers Y, Evangelista E, Lopez R, et al. Absence of γ-aminobutyric acid-a receptor potentiation in central hypersomnolence disorders. Ann Neurol 2016;80(2):259–68.

87. Trotti LM, Saini P, Bliwise DL, et al. Clarithromycin in γ-aminobutyric acid-Related hypersomnolence: a randomized, crossover trial. Ann Neurol 2015; 78(3):454–65.

88. Trotti LM, Saini P, Koola C, et al. Flumazenil for the treatment of refractory hypersomnolence: clinical experience with 153 patients. J Clin Sleep Med 2016;12(10):1389–94.

89. Miglis MG, Schneider L, Kim P, et al. Frequency and severity of autonomic symptoms in idiopathic hypersomnia. J Clin Sleep Med 2020;16(5):749–56.

90. Sforza E, Roche F, Barthélémy JC, et al. Diurnal and nocturnal cardiovascular variability and heart rate arousal response in idiopathic hypersomnia. Sleep Med 2016;24:131–6.

91. Materna L, Halfter H, Heidbreder A, et al. Idiopathic Hypersomnia Patients Revealed Longer Circadian Period Length in Peripheral Skin Fibroblasts. Front Neurol 2018;9:424.

92. Lippert J, Halfter H, Heidbreder A, et al. Altered dynamics in the circadian oscillation of clock genes in dermal fibroblasts of patients suffering from idiopathic hypersomnia. PLoS One 2014;9(1):e85255.

93. Fronczek R, Arnulf I, Baumann CR, et al. To split or to lump? Classifying the central disorders of hypersomnolence. Sleep 2020;(8).

94. Lopez R, Doukkali A, Barateau L, et al. Test-retest reliability of the multiple sleep latency test in central disorders of hypersomnolence. Sleep 2017;40(12).

95. Ruoff C, Pizza F, Trotti LM, et al. The MSLT is repeatable in narcolepsy type 1 but not narcolepsy type 2: a retrospective patient study. J Clin Sleep Med 2018;14(1):65–74.

96. Trotti LM, Staab BA, Rye DB. Test-retest reliability of the multiple sleep latency test in narcolepsy without cataplexy and idiopathic hypersomnia. J Clin Sleep Med 2013;9(8):789–95.

97. Pizza F, Barateau L, Jaussent I, et al. Validation of multiple sleep latency test for the diagnosis of pediatric narcolepsy type 1. Neurology 2019;93(11):e1034–44.

98. Diagnostic and statistical manual of mental disorders : DSM-5. Arlington, VA: American Psychiatric Association; 2013.

99. Krahn L.E., Arand D.L., Avidan A.Y., et al., Recommended protocols for the Multiple Sleep Latency Test and Maintenance of Wakefulness Test in adults: guidance from the American Academy of Sleep Medicine [published correction appears in J Clin Sleep Med. 2022 Aug 1;18(8):2089]. J Clin Sleep Med. 2021;17(12):2489-2498.

100. Wang Y-Q, Li R, Zhang M-Q, et al. The neurobiological mechanisms and treatments of REM sleep disturbances in depression. Curr Neuropharmacol 2015;13(4):543–53.

101. Wichniak A, Wierzbicka A, Jernajczyk W. Sleep as a biomarker for depression. Int Rev Psychiatry 2013;25(5):632–45.

102. Mansukhani MP, Dhankikar S, Kotagal S, et al. The influence of antidepressants and actigraphy-derived sleep characteristics on pediatric multiple sleep latency testing. J Clin Sleep Med 2021;17(11):2179–85.

103. Watson NF, Badr MS, Belenky G, et al. Recommended amount of sleep for a healthy adult: a joint consensus statement of the american academy of sleep medicine and sleep research society. Sleep 2015;38(6):843–4.

104. Dzodzomenyo S, Stolfi A, Splaingard D, et al. Urine toxicology screen in multiple sleep latency test: the correlation of positive tetrahydrocannabinol, drug negative patients, and narcolepsy. J Clin Sleep Med 2015;11(2):93–9.

105. Katz E, Maski K, Jenkins A. Drug testing in children with excessive daytime sleepiness during multiple sleep latency testing. J Clin Sleep Med 2014;10(8):897–901.

106. Vernet C, Arnulf I. Narcolepsy with long sleep time: a specific entity? Sleep 2009;32(9):1229–35.

107. Evangelista E, Lopez R, Barateau L, et al. Alternative diagnostic criteria for idiopathic hypersomnia: a 32-hour protocol. Ann Neurol 2018;83(2):235–47.

108. Cook JD, Eftekari SC, Leavitt LA, et al. Optimizing actigraphic estimation of sleep duration in suspected idiopathic hypersomnia. J Clin Sleep Med 2019;15(4):597–602.

109. Smith MT, McCrae CS, Cheung J, et al. Use of Actigraphy for the evaluation of sleep disorders and circadian rhythm sleep-wake disorders: an american academy of sleep medicine systematic review, meta-analysis, and GRADE assessment. J Clin Sleep Med 2018;14(7):1209–30.

110. Khosla S, Deak MC, Gault D, et al. Consumer sleep technology: an american academy of sleep medicine position statement. J Clin Sleep Med 2018;14(5):877–80.

111. Mignot E, Hayduk R, Black J, et al. HLA DQB1*0602 is associated with cataplexy in 509 narcoleptic patients. Sleep 1997;20(11):1012–20.

112. Capittini C, DeSilvestri A, Terzaghi M, et al. Correlation between HLA-DQB1*06:02 and narcolepsy with and without cataplexy: approving a safe and sensitive genetic test in four major ethnic groups. A systematic meta-analysis. Sleep Med 2018;52:150–7.

113. Coelho FMS, Pradella-Hallinan M, Neto MP, et al. Prevalence of the HLA-DQB1*0602 allele in narcolepsy and idiopathic hypersomnia patients seen at a sleep disorders outpatient unit in São Paulo. Br J Psychiatry 2009;31(1):10–4.

114. Barateau L, Lecendreux M, Chenini S, et al. Measurement of narcolepsy symptoms in school-aged children and adolescents: the pediatric narcolepsy severity scale. Neurology 2021;97(5):e476–88.

115. Dauvilliers Y, Evangelista E, Barateau L, et al. Measurement of symptoms in idiopathic hypersomnia: the idiopathic hypersomnia severity scale. Neurology 2019;92:e1754–62.

116. Maski K, Trotti LM, Kotagal S, et al. Treatment of central disorders of hypersomnolence: an American Academy of Sleep Medicine clinical practice guideline. J Clin Sleep Med 2021;17(9):1881–93.

117. Craig SG, Davies G, Schibuk L, et al. Long-term effects of stimulant treatment for ADHD: what can we tell our patients? Current Developmental Disorders Reports 2015;2:1–9.

118. Aran A, Einen M, Lin L, et al. Clinical and therapeutic aspects of childhood narcolepsy-cataplexy: a retrospective study of 51 children. Sleep 2010;33(11):1457–64.

119. Lecendreux M, Bruni O, Franco P, et al. Clinical experience suggests that modafinil is an effective and safe treatment for paediatric narcolepsy. J Sleep Res 2012;21(4):481–3.

120. Yeh S-B, Schenck CH. Efficacy of modafinil in 10 Taiwanese patients with narcolepsy: findings using the multiple sleep latency test and epworth sleepiness scale. Kaohsiung J Med Sci 2010;26(8):422–7.

121. Plazzi G, Ruoff C, Lecendreux M, et al. Treatment of paediatric narcolepsy with sodium oxybate: a double-blind, placebo-controlled, randomised-withdrawal multicentre study and open-label

investigation. Lancet Child & Adolescent Health 2018;2(7):483–94.

122. Black J, Reaven NL, Funk SE, et al. The Burden of Narcolepsy Disease (BOND) study: health-care utilization and cost findings. Sleep Med 2014;15(5):522–9.

123. Szakacs Z, Dauvilliers Y, Mikhaylov V, et al. Safety and efficacy of pitolisant on cataplexy in patients with narcolepsy: a randomised, double-blind, placebo-controlled trial. Lancet Neurol 2017;16(3):200–7.

124. Pullen LC, Picone Maria, Tan L, et al. Cognitive improvements in children with prader-willi syndrome following pitolisant treatment—patient reports. J Pediatr Pharmacol Therapeut 2019;24(2):166–71.

125. Baladi MG, Forster MJ, Gatch MB, et al. Characterization of the neurochemical and behavioral effects of solriamfetol (JZP-110), a selective dopamine and norepinephrine reuptake inhibitor. J Pharmacol Exp Ther 2018;366(2):367–76.

126. Thorpy MJ, Shapiro C, Mayer G, et al. A randomized study of solriamfetol for excessive sleepiness in narcolepsy. Ann Neurol 2019;85(3):359–70.

127. Vringer M, Kornum BR. Emerging therapeutic targets for narcolepsy. Expert Opin Ther Targets 2021;1–14. https://doi.org/10.1080/14728222.2021.1969361.

128. Dauvilliers Y, Arnulf I, Foldvary-Schaefer N, et al. Safety and efficacy of lower-sodium oxybate in adults with idiopathic hypersomnia: a phase 3, placebo-controlled, double-blind, randomised withdrawal study. Lancet Neurol 2022;21(1):53–65.

Restless Legs Syndrome and Restless Sleep Disorder in Children

Lourdes M. DelRosso, MD, PhD[a,b,*], Maria Paola Mogavero, MD[c,d,e], Oliviero Bruni, MD[f], Raffaele Ferri, MD[g]

KEYWORDS

- Restless legs syndrome • RLS • Restless sleep disorder • RSD • Iron supplementation • Ferritin

KEY POINTS

- Restless legs syndrome (RLS) is a clinical diagnosis and restless sleep disorder (RSD) requires polysomnography for diagnosis.
- RLS can present with symptoms of sleep onset or sleep maintenance insomnia while RSD presents with nonrestorative sleep.
- Both conditions are currently treated with iron supplementation.

RESTLESS LEGS SYNDROME

Restless legs syndrome (RLS) was first described in the 1600s by Thomas Willis as "tossing of the extremities," "restlessness," and insomnia and later on identified by Dr Ekbom in 1944 who described it in a case series of adult patients having "nocturnal paresthesia in the legs."[1] Since then, RLS has been recognized by the tetrad of "urge to move the legs," worsening of symptoms during rest, worsening of symptoms in the evening and improvement or resolution of symptoms after movement.[2] In children, RLS was also initially described by Dr Ekbom in 1975.[3] Later on, Walters and colleagues described a case series of 5 children with symptoms of RLS consisting of leg discomfort predominantly in the evening and relief with movement. Insomnia, restlessness, family history, and polysomnographic evidence of periodic limb movements during sleep (PLMS) are also contributing diagnostic features in children.[4]

DIAGNOSIS

The International RLS study group (IRLSSG) has published guidelines for the diagnosis of RLS in adults and children, stating the main difference in diagnosis is the fact that RLS symptoms in children must be expressed in the child's own words.[2] The diagnostic criteria in **Table 1** includes the key clinical components that can be obtained from the history and physical: urge to move the legs with worsening during evenings or quiescent period, improvement with movement, and not secondary to other conditions.

These criteria can be challenging to obtain in very young children or children, nonverbal or with syndromes or neurodevelopmental disorders. The American Academy of Sleep Medicine has published criteria for the use of polysomnography in nonrespiratory conditions and recommends that polysomnography can aid in the diagnosis of RLS because PLMS can be supportive of the

[a] University of California San Francisco, Fresno, USA; [b] University Sleep and Pulmonary Associates, 6733 North Willow Avenue, Unit 107, Fresno, CA 93710, USA; [c] Institute of Molecular Bioimaging and Physiology, National Research Council, Milan, Italy; [d] Division of Neuroscience, Sleep Disorders Center, San Raffaele Scientific Institute, Milan, Italy; [e] Centro di Medicina Del Sonno, IRCCS Ospedale San Raffaele, Turro, Via Stamira D'Ancona, 20, Milano 20127, Italy; [f] Department of Social and Developmental Psychology, Sapienza University, Via dei Marsi 78, Rome 00185, Italy; [g] Department of Neurology I.C., Sleep Research Centre, Oasi Research Institute - IRCCS, Via C Ruggero 73, Troina 94018, Italy
* Corresponding author. University of California San Francisco, University Sleep and Pulmonary Associates, 6733 North Willow Avenue, Unit 107, Fresno, CA 93710, USA.
E-mail address: lourdesdelrosso@me.com

Sleep Med Clin 18 (2023) 201–212
https://doi.org/10.1016/j.jsmc.2023.01.008
1556-407X/23/© 2023 Published by Elsevier Inc.

Table 1
Assessment tools available for pediatric restless legs syndrome

Validated in Adults and Utilized in Children	Specific to Pediatric RLS
• Single question for RLS • International RLS Severity Scale • Clinical Global Impressions Rating Scales • RLS-6 scale of Restless Legs Syndrome	• Pediatric Emory RLS Diagnostic Questionnaire • The Restless Legs Syndrome Questionnaire • Pediatric Restless Legs Syndrome Severity Scale

---

diagnosis.[5] A study on 103 children aged 2 to 19 years diagnosed with autism spectrum disorder and chronic insomnia showed that 39% were actually diagnosed with RLS. Leg kicking, body rocking, or restlessness in the legs was highly correlated with the diagnosis of RLS.[6] In this group, 77% of children with RLS had elevated PLMS on polysomnography (PSG), whereas those without RLS did not (mean PLMS 8.12 ± 6.59, range 0–26.1, $P < .0001$)[6] pointing out to a role for polysomnography in the diagnosis of RLS particularly when full criteria is not met due to the developmental stage of verbal abilities. Picchietti and colleagues found that 27 out of 69 children diagnosed with attention-deficit/hyperactivity disorder (ADHD) reported leg movements during sleep. A further polysomnographic study on these children showed that 18 out of 27 presented with a PLMS index above 5 per hour. Eight of these children had a family history of RLS. This evidence supports the interrelation between PLMS and RLS in children.[7]

A polysomnographic study assessing leg movements in children with RLS demonstrated important differences because school-aged children and adolescents. In fact the intermovement interval in children of school age showed a single peak between 2 and 4 seconds while in adolescents a second peak of 10 to 50 seconds is noted, close to that seen in adults.[8] Another important polysomnographic finding is that isolated leg movements may present earlier and disrupt sleep, months or years before the onset of RLS symptoms.[9]

Although there is some evidence for the use of actigraphy in the detection of PLMS in children with RLS (present in 80%),[10] there are currently no recommendations or guidelines for the use of actigraphy or activity monitors for the diagnosis of RLS. There are, however, some questionnaires that can be used for screening or severity assessment for Pediatric RLS[11] that are summarized in **Table 1** and discussed in the next section.

ASSESSMENT TOOLS OR QUESTIONNAIRES
Single Question for Restless Legs Syndrome

The single question incorporates the RLS diagnostic criteria elements: "when you try to relax in the evening or sleep at night, do you ever have unpleasant, restless feelings in your legs that can be relieved by walking or movement?"[12] and has been used in at least once epidemiology study of RLS in adolescents.[13] The single question shows a sensitivity of 100%, specificity of 96.8%, positive predictive value of 89.6%, and negative predictive value of 100%.

International Restless Legs Syndrome Severity Scale

The International RLS Severity Scale has been used in at least 6 studies involving children and adolescents.[14–18] It should be administered after a specific evaluation of symptoms and daytime function with the children and their parents.

Clinical Global Impressions Rating Scales

Clinical Global Impressions (CGI) Rating Scales are standard tools used in severity and change of clinical severity assessment for a very wide range of conditions; they are not specific to RLS. It has been used in a study specific to adolescents with RLS in at least one instance.[14] The CGI has also been used to assess improvement in symptoms after treatment with intravenous iron infusion.

Restless Legs Syndrome-6 Scale of Restless Legs Syndrome/Willis-Ekbom Disease

The RLS-6 has 6 items with a score from 0 to 10 for each of them; the symptoms are rated for their severity during the preceding week.[19] Items include severity of RLS at falling asleep and during the night, during the day (sitting or lying), and during the daytime activity. An additional item probes daytime sleepiness and last one assesses the patient satisfaction with his/her own sleep over the preceding 7 nights. At least one treatment study of RLS in adolescents used this scale.[14]

ASSESSMENT TOOLS SPECIFIC TO PEDIATRIC RESTLESS LEGS SYNDROME
Pediatric Emory Restless Legs Syndrome Diagnostic Questionnaire

The pediatric Emory RLS diagnostic questionnaire has 2 separate sets of questions for 2 different age groups age. For children aged 8 to 12 years, 47 questions need to be answered by the parent in the presence of the child. For adolescents aged 13 to 18 years, 46 questions can be answered by the subject. It has been used in children chronic kidney disease,[20] and in a separate study in children with nephrotic syndrome.[21] Unfortunately, this scale has not yet been fully validated.

The Restless Legs Syndrome Questionnaire

The Restless Legs Syndrome Questionnaire is a 11-item parent report questionnaire aiming at the assessment of pediatric RLS, developed after a literature review, interviews with parents, and a children's focus group.[22] The questionnaire has shown a 65% internal consistency and a repeated measure reliability with rho = 0.58. The original article reported no further details on the validation process and on the scale itself.

Pediatric Restless Legs Syndrome Severity Scale

The Pediatric Restless Legs Syndrome Severity Scale (P-RLS-SS) is a questionnaire with 41 Likert-type items based on a multicenter validation study during which children and adolescents aged 6 to 17 years were interviewed.[23] The P-RLS-SS assesses RLS symptoms and their impact on four domains: sleep, awake activities, emotions, and tiredness. The P-RLS-SS is a self-administered assessment tool and is recommended for children aged at least 9 years because younger children are likely to need assistance for completing it. However, P-RLS-SS is not yet validated.

Questionnaires are certainly valid tools, able to support the clinical assessment and diagnosis of pediatric RLS; however, the few scales available, which are specific for pediatric RLS, are not yet validated. Therefore, adult scales are currently used in adolescents with RLS because of their language ability. In younger subjects, it is still possible to use adult scales but only within a careful discussion of symptoms and daytime functioning with the children and their parents, in order to obtain a joint answer to each item.

EPIDEMIOLOGY

RLS affects approximately 2% to 4% of normally developing children and adolescents.[24] Pennestri and colleagues[25] used a questionnaire completed by the mother given at 7, 8, 12, 13, and 15 years, and found a prevalence between 2.4% and 3.1% between ages 7 and 15 years. At 12 years of age, the prevalence was higher in boys than in

girls. Another important finding was that when at least one parent was affected, the prevalence increased to 13.0%.[25] The prevalence can also be higher in specific populations at risk, for example, 22% of children with pediatric onset multiple sclerosis[26] and 11% of children with ADHD[27] have been diagnosed with RLS. In children with chronic kidney disease, the overall prevalence was 15.3% and did not vary depending on dialysis, transplant or nontransplant, nondialysis.[28]

The average age of symptom onset has been reported to be 10 to 11 years.[10] Although large percentages do not seek medical attention and can go undiagnosed for years.[10] A recent study assessing the prevalence on teenagers in Poland showed the presence of family history in 80% of cases, moderate symptoms in 61.9% of cases and intermittent course of symptoms in all of the cases.[10]

A study in schools in Turkey demonstrated that among children aged 9 to 18 years who fit diagnostic criteria for RLS, 65.6% were girls. In terms of symptom characteristics, 15.6% reported bilateral leg muscle pain, the urge to move the legs to relieve the unpleasant sensations was found in 39.3%, symptoms occurring at rest or when lying down were present in 36.4% and relief by gross movements was found in 21.4% of children.[29] Although leg pain or discomfort is expected in RLS, the urge to move legs can also be painless. In fact, a study in twins reported significantly higher correlations in monozygotic than in dizygotic twins only for the painful RLS subtype, whereas the painless RLS subtype was not genetically influenced but was independently associated with female sex (OR 0.52, $P = .003$) and iron deficiency (OR 4.20, $P < .001$).[30]

Excessive daytime sleepiness[26] and school problems are the most common daytime symptoms reported in children with RLS; however, other symptoms include disrupted sleep, behavioral problems (irritability, aggression, hyperactivity), attention deficit, and mood changes.

PATHOPHYSIOLOGY

The genetic contribution to RLS is widely accepted. To date there are greater than 20 loci identified to pose an increased risk for RLS.[31] The most widely studied genes are homeobox gene MEIS1, BTBD9, and LBXCOR1 on chromosomes 2p, 6p, and 15q, respectively, with MEIS1 being the strongest genetic risk factor for RLS. Each variant increased the risk of RLS by 50%.[32] Genetics in children has been found to be associated with the painful RLS subtype.[30] Usually

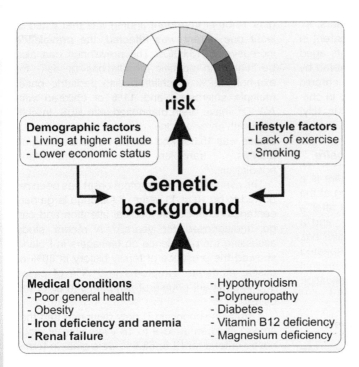

Fig. 1. The possible epigenetic risk factors of RLS interacting with its genetic background.

familial cases tend to present with symptoms at earlier age than nonfamiliar cases.[7,33]

Although very important, the genetic risk to develop RLS is clearly influenced by other demographic, lifestyle, socioeconomic, and health-related factors. However, it is difficult to assess the exact weight of these factors because it seems to be different in different individuals and studies assessing this type of risk are difficult to run.[34] **Fig. 1** provides a schematic representation of these possible epigenetic risk factors of RLS the discussion of which would be too extensive to be included in this article.

Iron deficiency is another contributor to the symptoms of RLS; 85% of children with RLS have been found to have blood levels of ferritin less than 50 ng/mL.[10] In children with chronic kidney disease, neither ferritin nor inflammation levels differ in children with RLS from children without RLS, suggesting a different pathophysiologic pathway in this group.[28]

The response to dopaminergic medications in RLS indicated, in previous studies, that brain dopaminergic neuronal pathways play a key role in this sleep-related movement disorder and, maybe, in other. Brain and spinal dopaminergic pathways postulated to be involved in RLS and PLMS include primarily a deficiency in the inhibitory A11 nucleus cell projections to the spinal cord, leading to increased sensory and motor activation, as well as increased sympathetic activity.[35]

The pathophysiology of low iron storages in RLS and PLMS has been studied in adults and autopsy studies have reported low brain iron storages in patients with RLS.[36] Moreover, MRI studies assessing regional brain iron content have confirmed low levels in the substantia nigra and putamen.[37] In addition, CSF ferritin has been shown to be low in patients with RLS, in particular in subjects in whom symptoms start at an age younger than 45 years.[38] Iron is a cofactor for tyrosine hydroxylase in the dopamine synthesis; therefore, low iron levels might be associated to low dopamine levels.

Other pathophysiological mechanisms have been proposed for RLS, such as the presence of a hyperglutamatergic state,[39,40] an altered level of brain adenosine,[41] or hypoxia.[42] The overall evidence supporting these alternatives to the dopaminergic hypothesis is lower and additional research is needed; however, it cannot be excluded that these different mechanisms can coexist and interact among themselves.

DIFFERENTIAL DIAGNOSIS

Growing pains usually affect children aged 4 to 6 years and occur intermittently in the evening, sparing the joints. The pain usually affects both legs, thighs and predominantly in the calf, and does not seem to be associated with erythema or swelling. Although some similarities exist between growing pains and RLS, the opposite does not apply because growing pains are not characterized by the urge to move the legs and the relief by movement.[43] The distinction between these 2 conditions in young children who do not understand "urge" but may identify RLS as a pain sensation is quite challenging. In this case, a careful evaluation, possibly supported by drawings and explanation of the symptoms in the child's own words may help differentiate both conditions.[44]

Painful nocturnal leg cramps can be also confused with RLS because they are alleviated by rubbing, massaging, or stretching the leg; however, the urge to move the legs is not present and they do not necessarily occur during rest/inactivity or in the evening before sleep.[45]

A study on children with ADHD and RLS symptoms found that 23% of 49 patients in their cohort had "mimics" of RLS that included myalgia (30/49), habitual foot tapping (23/49), positional discomfort (20/49), leg ulcer/bruise (1/49), and arthralgia/arthritis (1/49).[27]

Intuitively other musculoskeletal conditions found in children can also mimic leg discomfort include Osgood-Schlatter, acute injury, arthritis, connective tissue disorders, myopathy, sickle cell pain crisis, or neoplasms but these can be differentiated by tender points, inflammation, or abnormal radiographs.

Children with excessive motor activity during sleep can also be can be affected by a different condition called restless sleep disorder (RSD)[46] that has recently been identified in children with restless sleep and frequent movements or repositioning. However, these children do not have PLMS or other simple leg movement during sleep, and neither do they report the urge to move the legs nor there is family history of RLS.[47]

MANAGEMENT

Nonpharmacologic and pharmacologic treatments are available to manage RLS in children. The nonpharmacologic approaches involve sleep hygiene, diet control, and physical activity. Sleep hygiene refers to consistent activities and schedules around bedtime that promote sleep through appropriate environment and opportunity to sleep. General recommendations suggest to keep a cool temperature in the bedroom, comfortable mattress, and to avoid electronics at least for 1 hour before bedtime. The most important dietary modification is to avoid caffeinated products including coffee, tea, and chocolate after 3 PM[48] The last nonpharmacologic intervention is physical activity in the form of stretching exercises before bedtime. Stretching leg exercises have been reported to decrease symptoms of RLS,[49,50] probably by improving

circulation or by release of endorphins.[51] Rubbing or massaging the legs in children might help but no studies are available on this aspect.

There are no Food and Drug Administration (FDA)-approved medications for the treatment of RLS in children, thus drugs approved for adults are often used off-label. It is recommended that pharmacologic and nonpharmacologic treatments should always be combined, along with the elimination of factors that worsen or precipitate RLS and the evaluation of iron status.[52,53]

Similarly, the current guidelines[54] state that there is not enough evidence to recommend iron for RLS in children; nevertheless, most child sleep specialists do recommend supplementation with oral iron for children with RLS and serum ferritin levels less than 50 ng/mL.[55] Oral doses range between 3 and 6 mg/kg/d and may take 3 months or more to achieve relief of symptoms.[56] Some studies (generally open studies) have reported improvement of RLS symptoms after iron supplementation in children.[48,56–58] Only a single study is available on intravenous iron supplementation in children, reporting improvement in two-thirds of them.[59] Side effects include, more frequently, constipation and teeth staining, especially with liquid preparations.[60]

Alternative or add-on medications can be used in the case of insufficient response to iron supplementation, such as pramipexole[16]; however, only few data are available on the use of dopamine agonists in children with RLS.[14,61–68] This is important, also because dopaminergics are notorious for causing augmentation, sleepiness, insomnia, compulsive behaviors, and hallucinations; however, the impact of these side effects in children is not clear.

Gabapentin, another agent commonly used in adults with RLS, is known to be able to improve slow-wave sleep and sleep-onset latency.[69] In a small cohort of 2 children, gabapentin treatment led to the resolution of RLS symptoms.[48] Clonazepam, a long-acting benzodiazepine, is used in pediatric sleep medicine for the treatment of parasomnias. In adult RLS patients, it was able to improve sleep architecture and reduce arousals but did not modify PLMS RLS.[70,71] Finally, the alpha 2-adrenergic agonist clonidine is frequently used for insomnia and can be prescribed in combination with iron supplementation to improve sleep onset.[58] In adults, clonidine has been reported to reduce sensory manifestations of RLS.[72] No data are available on the utility of opioids in children.

RESTLESS SLEEP DISORDER

RSD is a recently identified pediatric sleep disorder characterized by a concern of restless sleep or frequent movements during sleep and significant daytime symptoms that are not explained by another condition. The current diagnostic criteria for RSD require polysomnography for diagnosis and include children aged from 6 to 18 years. Studies on RSD support iron deficiency, sleep instability, and increased sympathetic activation. RSD is more prevalent in children with ADHD and parasomnias. Expert taskforce consensus diagnostic criteria for RSD and for scoring large muscle group movements have been published. Iron supplementation has shown benefit improving sleep and daytime symptoms. Treatment options include iron supplementation either orally or intravenously.

DIAGNOSIS

Diagnostic criteria for RSD have been published. Symptoms must include parental concerns of restless sleep characterized by moving all night, trashing the bed, or having frequent body movements at night.[73] To fit full diagnostic criteria, RSD must be associated with daytime symptoms of fatigue, sleepiness, or behavioral problems.[73] When compared with children with RLS or normal controls, children with RSD do not show symptoms of insomnia such as difficulty falling asleep, nocturnal awakenings, leg discomfort, or leg movements on PSG.[73] Video polysomnography is required for the diagnosis and shows large muscle movement index of 5 or more.[74] Video PSG has also confirmed that children with RSD moved in their sleep frequently and through the whole night and every hour and through all sleep stages, which are likely to contribute to poor sleep quality and sleep disruption.[74]

Epworth Sleepiness Scale has shown scores greater than or equal to 10 comparable to children with RLS and periodic limb movement disorder (PLMD) but worse quality of life while compared with children with RLS and PLMD.[75] The authors also reported sleep architecture changes characterized by higher percentage of Rapid Eye Movement (REM), higher number of arousals, and increased percentage of wakefulness after sleep onset likely secondary to the frequent body movements and repositioning.[75] In another study with children with RSD and parasomnia, sleep efficiency was found to be more compromised in children with RSD and NREM parasomnias than in controls; cyclic alternating pattern (CAP), a marker of sleep instability was assessed[76] and found that subtypes A1, A2, and A3 were significantly increased in children with NREM parasomnias than in controls and subtype A3 was increased in children with RSD.[77]

EPIDEMIOLOGY

There are currently no studies assessing the prevalence of RSD in the general population. When studied in sleep clinic referred population, the prevalence was found to be 7.7%.[78] The prevalence among children with ADHD was found to be 9.1% although restless sleep was a common parental reported syndrome and a significant concern in 81.1% of children with ADHD. This may indicate that restlessness in children with ADHD is mainly secondary to other sleep disorders or comorbidities.[79] Recently, another study determines the prevalence of RSD in NREM sleep parasomnias to be 28.6%.[77]

PATHOPHYSIOLOGY

The underlying cause of RSD remains unknown but studies have tried to elucidate contributor to RSD. All evidence so far supports iron deficiency as a contributor. Studies have shown that children with RSD have a mean ferritin level of less than 20 ng/dL, which fits criteria for nonanemic iron deficiency, defined as ferritin levels less than 50 ng/dL. Low iron levels may alter dopaminergic pathways involved in motor activity.[80] Further support to iron deficiency contribution to RSD is the fact that sleep and daytime symptoms improve in children with RSD after iron supplementation.[81]

Movements during sleep could be secondary to sleep instability. Studies have analyzed a physiologic electroencephalographic marker of NREM sleep instability, called CAP found in polysomnography.[76] CAP has been studied and validated in children. Previous studies have shown an increased CAP rate in insomnia,[82] obstructive sleep apnea,[83,84] PLMD,[85] and seizures,[86] and decreased in narcolepsy.[87,88] Children with RSD have abnormal CAP findings, suggesting alterations in NREM sleep.[89] Particularly lower A3 subtypes, shorter duration of the B phase of the CAP cycle, and shorter CAP cycle were found in children with RSD when compared with controls. Large muscle movements in children with RSD occurred mainly during Non-CAP (NCAP) periods,[90] confirming that the movements are associated with significant sleep disruption.

Another hypothesis for the mechanism underlying RSD is an increase in sympathetic activity during sleep. Heart rate variability has been studied for many years in sleep medicine as marker of sympathetic/parasympathetic balance in sleep disorders.[91,92] In children with RSD, it showed a sympathetic predominance during sleep, whereas in children with RLS as expected, there was sympathetic predominance during the wakefulness period before sleep.[93,94]

Finally, spindle frequency, density, amplitude, and duration have been studied in association with developmental conditions, attention deficits and memory consolidation, demonstrating changes in spindle properties in children with neurodevelopmental disorders,[95–97] and children with sleep disorders.[98] The density of frontal spindles, especially during N2 sleep stage tended to decrease in children with RSD, compared with controls.[99,100]

DIFFERENTIAL DIAGNOSIS

The IRLSSG published a review of the differential diagnosis of restless sleep in children[101] identifying that many conditions presented with the subjective complaint of restless sleep complaint including obstructive sleep apnea,[102–104] RLS,[9,66,105–109] and PLMD.[110,111] Outside of the sleep medicine diagnosis, restless sleep was also seen in children with medical conditions such as acute otitis media,[112] asthma,[113–115] headaches, seizures,[116–119] eczema,[120] depression, anxiety,[121,122] and substance use such as caffeine.[123,124]

Due to the multiple conditions that can present with restless sleep, a diagnostic polysomnography is indicated for the objective diagnosis,[125] demonstrating at least 5 movements per hour during sleep.[46,73]

There are some tips to differentiate RSD from other sleep disorders. Children with RSD do not typically present with increased index of PLMS or bedtime symptoms of leg discomfort. They are not repetitive or stereotyped such as sleep-related rhythmic movement disorders, bruxism, and nocturnal epilepsy.[126] Body rocking or head rolling present usually at sleep onset or sleep stage transition,[127] and are clearly differentiated from RSD because the body movements and repositioning in RSD last through the night and do not follow a rhythmic or repetitive pattern. In bruxism, movements are confined to jaw clenching or teeth grinding, and these movements can result in arousals or awakenings.[128]

Even though the diagnosis of RSD is currently for children aged older than 6 years, we cannot ignore that RSD can exist before this age. However, at the current time, there is no criterion to diagnose RSD at this young age. The authors recommend to use a preliminary diagnosis of "insomnia with motor restlessness," check iron levels, supplement if recommended, and reassess.[129] Further studies are needed to define RSD in younger children.[129]

Management

The most intuitive treatment of RSD is iron supplementation due to the finding of low ferritin levels. So far, there are no other treatment options in the medical literature. Two publications support iron supplementation for treatment of RSD.[81,130] In one, oral iron supplementation was assessed,[81] and in the second one, oral iron supplementation with ferrous sulfate was compared with intravenous ferric carboxymaltose.[131] Oral iron was in the form of ferrous sulfate 325 mg tablet daily or liquid 3 mg/kg/d, and intravenous iron was ferric carboxymaltose in a single dose of 15 mg/kg if weight was less than 50 kg or a single dose of 750 mg if the weight was above 50 kg. Both groups showed subjective improvement in both daytime and nighttime symptoms and significant improvement in ferritin levels and iron profile.[130]

These results match those of other studies particularly in RLS, which have demonstrated symptomatic improvement after iron supplementation.[131] Because brain iron deficiency has been postulated to be a key factor in RLS, one can extrapolate that depending on the brain area affected, the phenotype or brain iron deficiency can manifest as RLS or RSD. Neuroimaging studies have demonstrated that brain iron deficiency in adult patients with RLS follows regional variations and specific locations such as the putamen and substantia nigra.[36,37,132] Transcranial ultrasound studies have shown improvement in iron stores in regions of the brainstem after intravenous iron infusion in adults with RLS.[133] Iron is a cofactor for dopamine production, and its deficiency may affect dopamine synthesis.[134] Imaging studies in children with RLS or RSD are still lacking.

SUMMARY

We have described the key features and recent findings on RLS and RSD in children. Poor sleep quality accounts for many consequences including daytime sleepiness, neurocognitive deficits, and medical comorbidities. Prompt identification and treatment of sleep-related movement disorders can prevent these consequences. Iron deficiency has been associated with both disorders and iron supplementation has improved both sleep and daytime symptoms.

CLINICS CARE POINTS

- Suspect RLS in children with leg discomfort and symptoms of insomnia.

- Suspect RSD in children with frequent movements during sleep and no other condition that can explain the sleep disturbance.
- Order PSG in children with suspicion of RSD but PSG is not needed for diagnosis of RLS.
- When diagnosing a child with RSD or RLS, order ferritin levels.
- In children with RSD or RLS and ferritin levels less than 50 ng/mL, consider supplementing iron with oral ferrous sulfate (3 mg/kg or single dose of 325 mg/d) or intravenous iron supplementation.

DECLARATION OF INTERESTS

The authors do not have any conflict of interest to disclose. There are no financial or nonfinancial disclosures.

REFERENCES

1. Ekbom KA. Asthenia Crurum Paraesthetica ("Irritable legs") A new syndrome consisting of weakeness, sensation of Cold and nocturnal paresthesia in the legs, responding to a Centain extent to treatment with Priscol and doryl.-A note on paresthesia in general. I Int Med 1944;118(1–3):197–209.
2. Allen RP, Picchietti DL, Garcia-Borreguero D, et al. Restless legs syndrome/Willis-Ekbom disease diagnostic criteria: updated International Restless Legs Syndrome Study Group (IRLSSG) consensus criteria–history, rationale, description, and significance. Sleep Med 2014;15(8):860–73.
3. Ekbom KA. Growing pains and restless legs. Acta Paediatr Scand 1975;64(2):264–6.
4. Walters AS, Picchietti DL, Ehrenberg BL, et al. Restless legs syndrome in childhood and adolescence. Pediatr Neurol 1994;11(3):241–5.
5. Kotagal S, Nichols CD, Grigg-Damberger MM, et al. Non-respiratory indications for polysomnography and related procedures in children: an evidence-based review. Sleep 2012;35(11):1451–66.
6. Kanney ML, Durmer JS, Trotti LM, et al. Rethinking bedtime resistance in children with autism: is restless legs syndrome to blame? J Clin Sleep Med 2020;16(12):2029–35.
7. Picchietti DL, England SJ, Walters AS, et al. Periodic limb movement disorder and restless legs syndrome in children with attention-deficit hyperactivity disorder. J Child Neurol 1998;13(12):588–94.
8. Ferri R, DelRosso LM, Arico D, et al. Leg movement activity during sleep in school-age children and adolescents: a detailed study in normal controls and

9. Picchietti DL, Stevens HE. Early manifestations of restless legs syndrome in childhood and adolescence. Sleep Med 2008;9(7):770–81.
10. Pienczk-Reclawowicz K, Pilarska E, Olszewska A, et al. The prevalence of the restless legs Syndrome/Willis-Ekbom disease among teenagers, its clinical characteristics and impact on everyday functioning. Sleep Med 2022;89:48–54.
11. Stubbs PH, Walters AS. Tools for the assessment of pediatric restless legs syndrome. Front Psychiatr 2020;11:356.
12. Ferri R, Lanuzza B, Cosentino FI, et al. A single question for the rapid screening of restless legs syndrome in the neurological clinical practice. Eur J Neurol 2007;14(9):1016–21.
13. Zhang J, Lam SP, Li SX, et al. Restless legs symptoms in adolescents: epidemiology, heritability, and pubertal effects. J Psychosom Res 2014;76(2):158–64.
14. Elshoff JP, Hudson J, Picchietti DL, et al. Pharmacokinetics of rotigotine transdermal system in adolescents with idiopathic restless legs syndrome (Willis-Ekbom disease). Sleep Med 2017;32:48–55.
15. Gagliano A, Arico I, Calarese T, et al. Restless Leg Syndrome in ADHD children: levetiracetam as a reasonable therapeutic option. Brain & development 2011;33(6):480–6.
16. Furudate N, Komada Y, Kobayashi M, et al. Daytime dysfunction in children with restless legs syndrome. J Neurol Sci 2014;336(1–2):232–6.
17. Bilgilisoy Filiz M, Filiz S, Baran RT, et al. Restless legs syndrome in children with allergic rhinitis: a comparative study on frequency, severity and sleep quality. Turkish journal of physical medicine and rehabilitation 2018;64(3):198–204.
18. Isikay S, Isikay N, Per H, et al. Restless leg syndrome in children with celiac disease. Turk J Pediatr 2018;60(1):70–5.
19. Kohnen R, Martinez-Martin P, Benes H, et al. Rating of daytime and nighttime symptoms in RLS: validation of the RLS-6 scale of restless legs syndrome/Willis-Ekbom disease. Sleep Med 2016;20:116–22.
20. Riar SK, Leu RM, Turner-Green TC, et al. Restless legs syndrome in children with chronic kidney disease. Pediatr Nephrol 2013;28(5):773–95.
21. Cheung V, Wertenteil S, Sasson S, et al. Restless legs syndrome in pediatric patients with nephrotic syndrome. Global pediatric health 2015;2. 2333794X15585994.
22. Evans A, Blunden S. Development of a parental report questionnaire for restless legs syndrome (RLS) in children: the RLSQ. J Foot Ankle Res 2011;4(1):O15.
23. Arbuckle R, Abetz L, Durmer JS, et al. Development of the pediatric restless legs syndrome

severity scale (P-RLS-SS): a patient-reported outcome measure of pediatric RLS symptoms and impact. Sleep Med 2010;11(9):897–906.

24. Picchietti D, Allen RP, Walters AS, et al. Restless legs syndrome: prevalence and impact in children and adolescents–the Peds REST study. Pediatrics 2007;120(2):253–66.

25. Pennestri MH, Petit D, Paquet J, et al. Childhood restless legs syndrome: a longitudinal study of prevalence and familial aggregation. J Sleep Res 2021;30(3):e13161.

26. Yalcinkaya BC, Amirov CB, Saltik S, et al. Restless legs syndrome in pediatric onset multiple sclerosis. Mult Scler Relat Disord 2021;56:103295.

27. Srifuengfung M, Bussaratid S, Ratta-Apha W, et al. Restless legs syndrome in children and adolescents with attention-deficit/hyperactivity disorder: prevalence, mimic conditions, risk factors, and association with functional impairment. Sleep Med 2020;73:117–24.

28. Riar SK, Greenbaum LA, Bliwise DL, et al. Restless legs syndrome in chronic kidney disease: is iron or inflammatory status to blame? J Clin Sleep Med 2019;15(11):1629–34.

29. Turkdogan D, Mahmudov R. Overlapping features of restless legs syndrome and growing pains in Turkish children and adolescents. Brain Dev 2022;44(6):372–9.

30. Champion D, Bui M, Aouad P, et al. Contrasting painless and painful phenotypes of pediatric restless legs syndrome: a twin family study. Sleep Med 2020;75:361–7.

31. Schormair B, Zhao C, Bell S, et al. Identification of novel risk loci for restless legs syndrome in genome-wide association studies in individuals of European ancestry: a meta-analysis. Lancet Neurol 2017;16(11):898–907.

32. Winkelmann J, Schormair B, Lichtner P, et al. Genome-wide association study of restless legs syndrome identifies common variants in three genomic regions. Nat Genet 2007;39(8):1000–6.

33. Lazzarini A, Walters AS, Hickey K, et al. Studies of penetrance and anticipation in five autosomal-dominant restless legs syndrome pedigrees. Mov Disord 1999;14(1):111–6.

34. Batool-Anwar S, Li Y, De VK, et al. Lifestyle factors and risk of restless legs syndrome: Prospective cohort study. J Clin Sleep Med 2015;jc–15.

35. Clemens S, Rye D, Hochman S. Restless legs syndrome: revisiting the dopamine hypothesis from the spinal cord perspective. Neurology 2006;67(1):125–30.

36. Connor JR, Boyer PJ, Menzies SL, et al. Neuropathological examination suggests impaired brain iron acquisition in restless legs syndrome. Neurology 2003;61(3):304–9.

37. Allen RP, Barker PB, Wehrl FW, et al. MRI measurement of brain iron in patients with restless legs syndrome. Neurology 2001;56(2):263–5.

38. Earley CJ, Connor JR, Beard JL, et al. Ferritin levels in the cerebrospinal fluid and restless legs syndrome: effects of different clinical phenotypes. Sleep 2005;28(9):1069–75.

39. Allen RP, Barker PB, Horska A, et al. Thalamic glutamate/glutamine in restless legs syndrome: increased and related to disturbed sleep. Neurology 2013;80(22):2028–34.

40. Ferre S, Garcia-Borreguero D, Allen RP, et al. New insights into the neurobiology of restless legs syndrome. Neuroscientist : a review journal bringing neurobiology, neurology and psychiatry 2019;25(2):113–25.

41. Ferre S. The adenosine hypothesis of restless legs syndrome. Journal of caffeine and adenosine research 2019;9(1):1–3.

42. Salminen AV, Rimpila V, Polo O. Peripheral hypoxia in restless legs syndrome (Willis-Ekbom disease). Neurology 2014;82(21):1856–61.

43. Walters AS, Gabelia D, Frauscher B. Restless legs syndrome (Willis-Ekbom disease) and growing pains: are they the same thing? A side-by-side comparison of the diagnostic criteria for both and recommendations for future research. Sleep Med 2013;14(12):1247–52.

44. Simakajornboon N, Dye TJ, Walters AS. Restless legs syndrome/willis-ekbom disease and growing pains in children and adolescents. Sleep Med Clin 2015;10(3):311–22, xiv.

45. Chokroverty S. Differential diagnoses of restless legs syndrome/willis-ekbom disease: mimics and comorbidities. Sleep Med Clin 2015;10(3):249–62, xii.

46. DelRosso LM, Ferri R, Allen RP, et al. Consensus diagnostic criteria for a newly defined pediatric sleep disorder: restless sleep disorder (RSD). Sleep Med 2020;75:335–40.

47. DelRosso LM, Jackson CV, Trotter K, et al. Video-polysomnographic characterization of sleep movements in children with restless sleep disorder. Sleep 2019;42(4).

48. Amos LB, Grekowicz ML, Kuhn EM, et al. Treatment of pediatric restless legs syndrome. Clinical pediatrics 2014;53(4):331–6.

49. Dinkins EM, Stevens-Lapsley J. Management of symptoms of Restless Legs Syndrome with use of a traction straight leg raise: a preliminary case series. Man Ther 2013;18(4):299–302.

50. Aukerman MM, Aukerman D, Bayard M, et al. Exercise and restless legs syndrome: a randomized controlled trial. J Am Board Fam Med 2006;19(5):487–93.

51. Bega D, Malkani R. Alternative treatment of restless legs syndrome: an overview of the evidence for

mind-body interventions, lifestyle interventions, and neutraceuticals. Sleep Med 2016;17:99–105.

52. Picchietti MA, Picchietti DL. Advances in pediatric restless legs syndrome: iron, genetics, diagnosis and treatment. Sleep Med 2010;11(7):643–51.

53. Garcia-Borreguero D, Kohnen R, Silber MH, et al. The long-term treatment of restless legs syndrome/Willis-Ekbom disease: evidence-based guidelines and clinical consensus best practice guidance: a report from the International Restless Legs Syndrome Study Group. Sleep Med 2013; 14(7):675–84.

54. Allen RP, Picchietti DL, Auerbach M, et al. Evidence-based and consensus clinical practice guidelines for the iron treatment of restless legs syndrome/Willis-Ekbom disease in adults and children: an IRLSSG task force report. Sleep Med 2018;41:27–44.

55. Earley CJ. Clinical practice. Restless legs syndrome. N Engl J Med 2003;348(21):2103–9.

56. Mohri I, Kato-Nishimura K, Kagitani-Shimono K, et al. Evaluation of oral iron treatment in pediatric restless legs syndrome (RLS). Sleep Med 2012; 13(4):429–32.

57. Tilma J, Tilma K, Norregaard O, et al. Early childhood-onset restless legs syndrome: symptoms and effect of oral iron treatment. Acta paediatrica 2013;102(5):e221–6.

58. Dye TJ, Jain SV, Simakajornboon N. Outcomes of long-term iron supplementation in pediatric restless legs syndrome/periodic limb movement disorder (RLS/PLMD). Sleep Med 2017;32:213–9.

59. Grim K, Lee B, Sung AY, et al. Treatment of childhood-onset restless legs syndrome and periodic limb movement disorder using intravenous iron sucrose. Sleep Med 2013;14(11):1100–4.

60. Picchietti DL. Should oral iron be first-line therapy for pediatric restless legs syndrome and periodic limb movement disorder? Sleep Med 2017;32: 220–1.

61. Walters AS, Mandelbaum DE, Lewin DS, et al. Dopaminergic therapy in children with restless legs/periodic limb movements in sleep and ADHD. Dopaminergic Therapy Study Group. Pediatr Neurol 2000;22(3):182–6.

62. Konofal E, Arnulf I, Lecendreux M, et al. Ropinirole in a child with attention-deficit hyperactivity disorder and restless legs syndrome. Pediatr Neurol 2005;32(5):350–1.

63. Kotagal S, Silber MH. Childhood-onset restless legs syndrome. Ann Neurol 2004;56(6):803–7.

64. Muhle H, Neumann A, Lohmann-Hedrich K, et al. Childhood-onset restless legs syndrome: clinical and genetic features of 22 families. Mov Disord : official journal of the Movement Disorder Society 2008;23(8):1113–21. quiz 1203.

65. Starn AL, Udall JN Jr. Iron deficiency anemia, pica, and restless legs syndrome in a teenage girl. Clinical pediatrics 2008;47(1):83–5.

66. Picchietti DL, Walters AS. Moderate to severe periodic limb movement disorder in childhood and adolescence. Sleep 1999;22(3):297–300.

67. England SJ, Picchietti DL, Couvadelli BV, et al. L-Dopa improves Restless Legs Syndrome and periodic limb movements in sleep but not Attention-Deficit-Hyperactivity Disorder in a double-blind trial in children. Sleep Med 2011;12(5):471–7.

68. Cortese S, Konofal E, Lecendreux M. Effectiveness of ropinirole for RLS and depressive symptoms in an 11-year-old girl. Sleep Med 2009; 10(2):259–61.

69. Foldvary-Schaefer N, De Leon Sanchez I, Karafa M, et al. Gabapentin increases slow-wave sleep in normal adults. Epilepsia 2002;43(12): 1493–7.

70. Saletu M, Anderer P, Saletu-Zyhlarz GM, et al. Comparative placebo-controlled polysomnographic and psychometric studies on the acute effects of gabapentin versus ropinirole in restless legs syndrome. Journal of neural transmission 2010;117(4):463–73.

71. Manconi M, Ferri R, Zucconi M, et al. Dissociation of periodic leg movements from arousals in restless legs syndrome. Ann Neurol 2012;71(6):834–44.

72. Prince JB, Wilens TE, Biederman J, et al. Clonidine for sleep disturbances associated with attention-deficit hyperactivity disorder: a systematic chart review of 62 cases. J Am Acad Child Adolesc Psychiatry 1996;35(5):599–605.

73. DelRosso LM, Bruni O, Ferri R. Restless sleep disorder in children: a pilot study on a tentative new diagnostic category. Sleep 2018;41(8):zsy102.

74. DelRosso LM, Jackson CV, Trotter K, et al. Video-polysomnographic characterization of sleep movements in children with restless sleep disorder. Sleep 2019;42(4):zsy269.

75. Liu WK, Dye TJ, Horn P, et al. Large body movements on video-polysomnography are associated with daytime dysfunction in children with restless sleep disorder. Sleep 2022;45(4):zsac005.

76. Parrino L, Ferri R, Bruni O, et al. Cyclic alternating pattern (CAP): the marker of sleep instability. Sleep Med Rev 2012;16(1):27–45.

77. Senel GB, Kochan Kizilkilic E, Karadeniz D. Restless sleep disorder in children with NREM parasomnias. Sleep 2021;44(7).

78. DelRosso LM, Ferri R. The prevalence of restless sleep disorder among a clinical sample of children and adolescents referred to a sleep centre. J Sleep Res 2019;28(6):e12870.

79. Kapoor V, Ferri R, Stein MA, et al. Restless sleep disorder in children with attention-deficit/

hyperactivity disorder. J Clin Sleep Med 2021; 17(4):639–43.

80. Angulo-Barroso RM, Peirano P, Algarin C, et al. Motor activity and intra-individual variability according to sleep-wake states in preschool-aged children with iron-deficiency anemia in infancy. Early Hum Dev 2013;89(12):1025–31.

81. DelRosso LM, Yi T, Chan JHM, et al. Determinants of ferritin response to oral iron supplementation in children with sleep movement disorders. Sleep 2020;43(3):zsz234.

82. Terzano MG, Parrino L. Evaluation of EEG cyclic alternating pattern during sleep in insomniacs and controls under placebo and acute treatment with zolpidem. Sleep 1992;15(1):64–70.

83. Hartmann S, Bruni O, Ferri R, et al. Cyclic alternating pattern in children with obstructive sleep apnea and its relationship with adenotonsillectomy, behavior, cognition, and quality of life. Sleep 2021;44(1).

84. Gnoni V, Drakatos P, Higgins S, et al. Cyclic alternating pattern in obstructive sleep apnea: a preliminary study. J Sleep Res 2021;e13350.

85. Parrino L, Boselli M, Buccino GP, et al. The cyclic alternating pattern plays a gate-control on periodic limb movements during non-rapid eye movement sleep. J Clin Neurophysiol 1996;13(4):314–23.

86. Zucconi M, Oldani A, Smirne S, et al. The macro-structure and microstructure of sleep in patients with autosomal dominant nocturnal frontal lobe epilepsy. J Clin Neurophysiol 2000;17(1):77–86.

87. Ferri R, Miano S, Bruni O, et al. NREM sleep alterations in narcolepsy/cataplexy. Clinical neurophysiology : official journal of the International Federation of Clinical Neurophysiology 2005; 116(11):2675–84.

88. Ferri R, Franceschini C, Zucconi M, et al. Sleep polygraphic study of children and adolescents with narcolepsy/cataplexy. Dev Neuropsychol 2009;34(5):523–38.

89. DelRosso LM, Hartmann S, Baumert M, et al. Non-REM sleep instability in children with restless sleep disorder. Sleep Med 2020;75:276–81.

90. Parrino L, Smerieri A, Rossi M, et al. Relationship of slow and rapid EEG components of CAP to ASDA arousals in normal sleep. Sleep 2001;24(8):881–5.

91. Stein PK, Pu Y. Heart rate variability, sleep and sleep disorders. Sleep Med Rev 2012;16(1):47–66.

92. Martin-Montero A, Gutierrez-Tobal GC, Kheirandish-Gozal L, et al. Heart rate variability spectrum characteristics in children with sleep apnea. Pediatr Res 2021;89(7):1771–9.

93. Ferri R, Parrino L, Smerieri A, et al. Cyclic alternating pattern and spectral analysis of heart rate variability during normal sleep. J Sleep Res 2000; 9(1):13–8.

94. Snyder F, Hobson JA, Morrison DF, et al. Changes in respiration, heart rate, and systolic blood Pressure in human sleep. J Appl Physiol 1964;19: 417–22.

95. Gruber R, Wise MS. Sleep spindle characteristics in children with neurodevelopmental disorders and their relation to cognition. Neural Plast 2016; 2016:4724792.

96. Bruni O, Ferri R, Novelli L, et al. Sleep spindle activity is correlated with reading abilities in developmental dyslexia. Sleep 2009;32(10):1333–40.

97. Saito Y, Kaga Y, Nakagawa E, et al. Association of inattention with slow-spindle density in sleep EEG of children with attention deficit-hyperactivity disorder. Brain Dev 2019;41(9):751–9.

98. Brockmann PE, Damiani F, Pincheira E, et al. Sleep spindle activity in children with obstructive sleep apnea as a marker of neurocognitive performance: a pilot study. Eur J Paediatr Neurol : EJPN : official journal of the European Paediatric Neurology Society 2018;22(3):434–9.

99. DelRosso LM, Mogavero MP, Brockmann P, et al. Sleep spindles in children with restless sleep disorder, restless legs syndrome and normal controls. Clinical neurophysiology : official journal of the International Federation of Clinical Neurophysiology 2021;132(6):1221–5.

100. O'Reilly C, Nielsen T. Assessing EEG sleep spindle propagation. Part 2: experimental characterization. J Neurosci Methods 2014;221:215–27.

101. DelRosso LM, Picchietti DL, Spruyt K, et al. Restless sleep in children: a systematic review. Sleep Med Rev 2021;56:101406.

102. Brouilette R, Hanson D, David R, et al. A diagnostic approach to suspected obstructive sleep apnea in children. J Pediatr 1984;105(1):10–4.

103. Martha VF, Moreira Jda S, Martha AS, et al. Reversal of pulmonary hypertension in children after adenoidectomy or adenotonsillectomy. Int J Pediatr Otorhinolaryngol 2013;77(2):237–40.

104. Sakellaropoulou AV, Hatzistilianou MN, Emporiadou MN, et al. Association between primary nocturnal enuresis and habitual snoring in children with obstructive sleep apnoea-hypopnoea syndrome. Arch Med Sci 2012;8(3): 521–7.

105. Rosen GM, Morrissette S, Larson A, et al. Does improvement of low serum ferritin improve symptoms of restless legs syndrome in a cohort of pediatric patients? J Clin Sleep Med : JCSM : official publication of the American Academy of Sleep Medicine 2019;15(8):1149–54.

106. Gingras JL, Gaultney JF, Picchietti DL. Pediatric periodic limb movement disorder: sleep symptom and polysomnographic correlates compared to obstructive sleep apnea. J Clin Sleep Med :

JCSM : official publication of the American Academy of Sleep Medicine 2011;7(6):603–609A.

107. Turkdogan D, Bekiroglu N, Zaimoglu S. A prevalence study of restless legs syndrome in Turkish children and adolescents. Sleep Med 2011;12(4):315–21.

108. Yilmaz K, Kilincaslan A, Aydin N, et al. Prevalence and correlates of restless legs syndrome in adolescents. Dev Med Child Neurol 2011;53(1):40–7.

109. Picchietti DL, Rajendran RR, Wilson MP, et al. Pediatric restless legs syndrome and periodic limb movement disorder: parent-child pairs. Sleep Med 2009;10(8):925–31.

110. Walter LM, Nixon GM, Davey MJ, et al. Differential effects of sleep disordered breathing on polysomnographic characteristics in preschool and school aged children. Sleep Med 2012;13(7):810–5.

111. American Academy of Sleep Medicine. International classification of sleep disorders. 3rd ed. Darien, IL: American Academy of Sleep Medicine.; 2014.

112. Uitti JM, Salanterä S, Laine MK, et al. Adaptation of pain scales for parent observation: are pain scales and symptoms useful in detecting pain of young children with the suspicion of acute otitis media? BMC Pediatr 2018;18(1):392.

113. Meltzer LJ, Pugliese CE. Sleep in young children with asthma and their parents. J Child Health Care : for professionals working with children in the hospital and community 2017;21(3):301–11.

114. Verhulst SL, Vekemans K, Ho E, et al. Is wheezing associated with decreased sleep quality in Sri Lankan children? A questionnaire study. Pediatr Pulmonol 2007;42(7):579–83.

115. Desager KN, Nelen V, Weyler JJ, et al. Sleep disturbance and daytime symptoms in wheezing school-aged children. J Sleep Res 2005;14(1):77–82.

116. Esin OR. Treatment of tension-type headaches in adolescents (14–15 Years old): the efficacy of aminophenylbutyric acid hydrochloride. BioNanoScience 2018;8(1):418–22.

117. Becker DA, Fennell EB, Carney PR. Sleep disturbance in children with epilepsy. Epilepsy Behav 2003;4(6):651–8.

118. Bruni O, Galli F, Guidetti V. Sleep hygiene and migraine in children and adolescents. Cephalalgia : an international journal of headache 1999; 19(Suppl 25):57–9.

119. Wang X, Marcuse LV, Jin L, et al. Sleep-related hypermotor epilepsy activated by rapid eye movement sleep. Epileptic Disord 2018;20(1):65–9.

120. Camfferman D, Kennedy JD, Gold M, et al. Sleep and neurocognitive functioning in children with eczema. Int J Psychophysiol 2013;89(2):265–72.

121. Ivanenko A, Crabtree VM, Obrien LM, et al. Sleep complaints and psychiatric symptoms in children evaluated at a pediatric mental health clinic. J Clin Sleep Med 2006;2(1):42–8.

122. Mehl RC, O'Brien LM, Jones JH, et al. Correlates of sleep and pediatric bipolar disorder. Sleep 2006; 29(2):193–7.

123. Watson EJ, Banks S, Coates AM, et al. The relationship between caffeine, sleep, and behavior in children. J Clin Sleep Med 2017;13(4):533–43.

124. DelRosso L, Bruni O. Treatment of pediatric restless legs syndrome. Adv Pharmacol 2019;84: 237–53.

125. Berry RBBR, Gramaldo CE, et al. For the American Academy of sleep medicine. The AASM Manual for the scoring of sleep and associated Events, 2.4. Darien, Illinois: AASM; 2017.

126. Vendrame M, Kothare SV. Epileptic and nonepileptic paroxysmal events out of sleep in children. J Clin Neurophysiol 2011;28(2):111–9.

127. DelRosso LM, Mogavero MP, Ferri R. Restless sleep disorder, restless legs syndrome, and periodic limb movement disorder-Sleep in motion! Pediatr Pulmonol 2021;57(8):1879–86.

128. Alfano CA, Bower JL, Meers JM. Polysomnography-Detected bruxism in children is associated with somatic complaints but not anxiety. J Clin Sleep Med 2018;14(1):23–9.

129. Bruni O, Sette S, Angriman M, et al. Clinically oriented subtyping of chronic insomnia of childhood. J Pediatr 2018;196:194–200 e191.

130. DelRosso LM, Picchietti DL, Ferri R. Comparison between oral ferrous sulfate and intravenous ferric carboxymaltose in children with restless sleep disorder. Sleep 2021;44(2).

131. Wang J, O'Reilly B, Venkataraman R, et al. Efficacy of oral iron in patients with restless legs syndrome and a low-normal ferritin: a randomized, double-blind, placebo-controlled study. Sleep Med 2009; 10(9):973–5.

132. Rizzo G, Manners D, Testa C, et al. Low brain iron content in idiopathic restless legs syndrome patients detected by phase imaging. Mov Disord 2013;28(13):1886–90.

133. Garcia-Malo C, Wanner V, Miranda C, et al. Quantitative transcranial sonography of the substantia nigra as a predictor of therapeutic response to intravenous iron therapy in restless legs syndrome. Sleep Med 2019;66:123–9.

134. Allen RP. Restless leg syndrome/willis-ekbom disease pathophysiology. Sleep Med Clin 2015; 10(3):207–14, xi.

Sleep and Inflammation
Bidirectional Relationship

Haviva Veler, MD

KEYWORDS

- Sleep • Inflammation • Interleukin-6 • Tumor necrosis factor • C-reactive protein

KEY POINTS

- There is a bidirectional relationship between sleep and inflammation, where certain inflammatory markers follow circadian rhythms and show fluctuation in their blood levels depending on the time of day. In turn, pro-inflammatory cytokines, such as interleukin-1 (IL-1) and tumor necrosis factor (TNF), have been shown to modulate physiologic sleep.
- Many cytokines and chemokines have been studied in laboratory animals or human subjects and were shown to affect sleep. Of these, the most extensively studied inflammatory cytokines in sleep regulation are IL-1β, IL-6, and TNF-α.
- Inflammatory cytokines are the connecting line between the different morbidities seen in subjects with insufficient sleep, either as part of sleep apnea syndromes or insomnia.
- Insufficient as well as irregular sleep can lead to increased inflammation, as reflected by elevated levels of C-reactive protein. Therefore, improved sleep hygiene and implementation of appropriate sleep schedule can decrease inflammation.

INTRODUCTION

Sleep has a dynamic role in regulating major effector systems of the central nerve system (CNS), such as the hypothalamic–pituitary–adrenal (HPA) and the sympathetic nervous system (SNS), and the immune system. During nocturnal normal sleep in humans, both sleep and the circadian oscillator influence inflammatory activity.[1] It is widely established that sleep plays an important role in recovery from infectious disease and even in the folklore it is believed that increased sleep during infection is protective. This is mediated by antimicrobial peptides and cytokines that cause lethargy and enhance sleep.[2]

Circadian Rhythmicity of Inflammatory Cytokines During Normal sleep

Certain inflammatory markers follow circadian rhythms and show fluctuation in their blood levels depending on the time of day. For example, interleukin-6 (IL-6) is a pro-inflammatory cytokine with effect on inflammation, immune response, and hematopoiesis. Systemic levels of IL-6 have a circadian profile with peaks at 7 PM and 5 AM. Nocturnal sleep is necessary for the nocturnal increases in IL-6 levels and in addition for the production of tumor necrosis factor (TNF) by stimulated monocytes.[3] Experimental sleep deprivation induces an under secretion of IL-6 during the nocturnal period, delays the nocturnal increase of IL-6 levels, and attenuates monocyte production of TNF during the night. Sleep deprivation shifts the pattern of IL-6 secretion from nighttime to daytime, leading to an oversecretion of IL-6 during the day.[4] Interestingly, higher levels of IL-6 occur during REM sleep.

The CNS regulates two main effector systems that mediate changes in inflammatory responses during sleep and in response to sleep disturbance. When the HPA axis is activated the glucocorticoid cortisol is released, which is a potent anti-inflammatory mediator. In contrary, the SNS favors activation of the inflammatory response accompanying the downregulation of antiviral immune responses. SNS-mediated effects on innate

Pediatric Pulmonology and Sleep Medicine, University of Connecticut School of Medicine, Connecticut Children Medical Center, 85 Seymour Street, Suite 500, Hartford, CT 06106, USA
E-mail address: hveler@connecticutchildren.org

Sleep Med Clin 18 (2023) 213–218
https://doi.org/10.1016/j.jsmc.2023.02.003
1556-407X/23/© 2023 Published by Elsevier Inc.

immune response involve the suppression of type I interferon-mediated antiviral responses and the upregulation of transcription of inflammatory cytokine genes, such as those encoding IL-1β, TNF, and IL-6.[1]

Other immune-mediated changes that take place during normal sleep include antigen-presenting cells and T cells are redistributed from the circulation and accumulate in lymphoid tissue.[5] In addition, sleep promotes the activation of T cells through their increased production of IL-2 and IFNγ, as well as the production of IL-12 by dendritic cells and monocytes, which has a crucial role in inducing T helper type 1 (TH1) cell-type adaptive immune responses. During the night, there is a sleep-related shift toward TH1 cell-type immune responses, with increased expression of IFNγ by T cells and decreased expression of the anti-inflammatory cytokine IL-10 by monocytes.[1]

Inflammatory cytokine's effect on sleep

Pro-inflammatory cytokines, such as IL-1 and TNF, have been shown to modulate physiologic sleep. Plasma IL-1β concentration is highest at the onset of sleep in humans suggesting a sleep wake cycle variation of this cytokine. Cloned IL-1 receptor antagonist transiently inhibits non-REM (rapid eye movements) (NREM) sleep in rabbits. Substances that promote IL-1β production, such as endotoxin and TNF-α, enhance NREM sleep, and materials that inhibit its production, such as prostaglandin E2 and corticosteroids, inhibit sleep. Elevated plasma TNF-α levels are associated with enhanced slow wave amplitudes during sleep. In rabbits given a fragment of TNF-α soluble receptor, spontaneous NREM sleep was suppressed by 40%.[6]

Pro-Inflammatory Cytokines and Obstructive Sleep Apnea Syndrome

In adults

Vgontzas and colleagues[7] determined plasma levels of IL-1β, TNF-α, and IL-6 in patients with obstructive sleep apnea syndrome (OSAS) and hypersomnia in comparison to control subjects. The concentration of TNF-α was significantly elevated in patients with OSAS and correlated with the intensity of sleepiness measured as mean nap sleep latency. IL-6 levels were elevated only in OSAS and correlated with body mass index. The same investigators also found that the concentrations of IL-6 and TNF-α were higher in obese men with OSAS compared with non-apneic obese men; therefore, OSAS is likely associated with elevated plasma concentrations of IL-6 and TNF-α independent of obesity.[6] In OSAS

models, both in vivo and ex vivo, the normal nocturnal peak was absent and an additional daytime peak had developed. Considering the elevated systemic levels of TNF-α correlates with induced sleepiness in humans and muscle weakness in laboratory animals,[8] it is speculated that it is responsible to the clinical symptomatology of OSAS.

Systemic inflammation is usually measured by levels of C-reactive proteins (CRP). An elevated plasma level of this acute phase reactant indicates heightened activity of inflammation in humans. The presence of elevated CRP levels is also associated with increased risk of cardiovascular and cerebrovascular mortality. CRP is elevated in a number of inflammatory states, in regard to sleep, it was independently elevated in adults with obesity, even after controlling for comorbid conditions, such as inflammatory diseases, cardiovascular disease, and diabetes mellitus.[9] In addition, CRP levels are elevated in adults with OSAS and even more were independently associated with severity of sleep-disordered breathing. Yokoe and colleagues compared the levels of CRP and IL-6 in 30 men with newly diagnosed OSAS against a control group of 14 obese men before and after nasal CPAP therapy.[10] Monocyte production of IL-6, serum levels of IL-6, and CRP were elevated in patients with OSAS compared with obese control subjects. One month of nasal CPAP therapy was associated with marked reduction in serum levels and monocyte production of IL-6 and CRP. As body mass index (BMI) did not change in these patients, the author concluded that these findings are independent of weight. In addition, IL-6 levels were independently associated with nocturnal hypoxia suggesting hypoxia-primed monocytes as the source of the rise.

Other marker for systemic inflammation is leptin. Leptin is an adipocyte-derived hormone that reduces appetite, increases energy expenditure, and decreases body weight. It is also pleiotropic hormone that has immunomodulatory properties including enhancement of phagocytic function, stimulation of memory T-cell maturation, and certain anti-inflammatory properties. Ip and colleagues[11] showed that patients with OSAS had significantly higher serum levels of leptin compared with BMI-matched controls. Following treatment with nasal continous positive airway pressure (CPAP) for 6 months, there was a significant reduction in leptin levels in the absence of any change in BMI.

In adults, the inflammatory cascade described was suggested as a contributor to anatomic upper airway narrowing, abnormalities in upper airway reflexes, upper airway collapsibility, and inspiratory pharyngeal muscle dysfunction. These unfavorable processes may increase the severity of OSAS, setting up a vicious cycle. Activation of neutrophils and monocytes and elaboration of pro-inflammatory cytokines, TNF-α and IL-6 in particular, could play a role in the pathogenesis of OSAS. The symptoms of lethargy and excessive daytime hyper somnolence may be mediated, in part, by these processes.[6]

In children

The concept linking inflammation and pediatric OSAS was initially invoked by Tauman and colleagues in 2004.[12] Then, the presence of chronic low-grade inflammation was known to be present in children, but whether the inflammatory mechanisms were a component or the cause of this syndrome was not clear. Since then, a large body of research was done and confirmed the association, particularly when concurrent obesity, another chronic low-grade inflammatory disorder, is present.

General Inflammatory Concepts

The initial activation of the innate immune system response is done by the toll-like receptors (TLRs), an important family of receptors that constitute the first line of defense system. They can recognize both invading pathogens and endogenous danger molecules and are widely distributed in both immune and other body cells. TLRs induce the production of inflammatory cytokines (eg, TNF-α, IL-1, and IL-6) and chemokines (eg, CCL2 and CXCL8) as well as prostaglandins. Interestingly, sleep deprivation alone can lead to stimulation of the TLR pathways and induce cytokine production.[13]

NF-kB, an important transcription factor underlying the activation and regulation of inflammatory pathways, is involved in the transcription of genes responsible for the production of cytokines and inflammatory markers.[14] Sleep deprivation, even mild, can induce the activation and translocation of NF-kB in specific brain regions associated with sleep regulation, which lead to localized inflammatory responses. The list of cytokines and chemokines that has been studied in laboratory animals or human subjects and demonstrated to affect sleep is quite substantial.[15] Of these, the most extensively studied inflammatory cytokines in sleep regulation are IL-1β, IL-6, and TNF-α and these will be discussed in this summary.

Inflammation and Obesity

Adipose tissue produces a host of chemokines, termed adipokines, with well-described effects on metabolism and inflammation. Resistin, adiponectin, leptin, and monocyte chemoattractant protein-1 (MCP-1) are among a group of secreted proteins from adipose tissue which exhibit immunomodulatory functions.[16] Obesity is a pro-inflammatory state, where secretion of MCP-1, resistin, and other pro-inflammatory cytokines is increased and in turn the anti-inflammatory protein adiponectin is decreased.[17]

Another element contributing the inflammatory response in obesity is the adipocyte-infiltrated macrophages, which are highly inflammatory and, up activation, will secrete a wide variety of pro-inflammatory proteins including MCP-1, TNF-α, and IL-6.18

Another mechanism involves alterations in hormones that regulate appetite. Adipocytes produce leptin that is a member of the adipokine family. It is widely accepted that leptin can directly link nutritional status and pro-inflammatory T-helper 1 immune responses and that a decrease of leptin plasma concentration during food deprivation can lead to an impaired immune function. In addition, several studies have implicated leptin in the pathogenesis of chronic inflammation, and the elevated circulating leptin levels in obesity seem to contribute to the low-grade inflammatory background, which makes obese individuals more susceptible to the increased risk of developing cardiovascular diseases, type II diabetes, or degenerative disease including autoimmunity and cancer.[19]

Inflammatory Mechanisms in Cardiovascular Complications of Obstructive Sleep Apnea Syndrome

OSAS exposes the cardiovascular system to intermittent hypoxia and increased recurring negative intrathoracic pressures as well as to sleep fragmentation and therefore triggers increased sympathetic hyperactivity and inflammation. OSAS has been shown to promote atherosclerosis via the formation and release of cytokines including IL-1, IL-6, TNF-α, and other adipokines from adipose tissues and circulating inflammatory cell.[20] Increased inflammation will further the production and release of acute phase reactants such as CRP from the liver, which in turn will induce substantial endothelial dysfunction possibly via oxidative stress.[13] All these events will promote increased expression of adhesion molecules leading to activation of platelets and other procoagulant factors.[21]

In adults, TNF-α is a well-established pro-inflammatory cytokine that is involved in atherosclerosis by inducing the expression of cellular adhesion molecules that mediate the leukocyte adhesion to the vascular endothelium.[22] In children, a large prospective study from Gozal and colleagues included 298 children and showed that morning levels of TNF-α were increased in the presence of OSAS, particularly in the more severe cases and that these levels decreased after adenotonsillectomy (AT).[23] Furthermore, TNF-α levels were strongly associated with the degree of respiratory-induced sleep fragmentation.

CRP, as a well-known marker of inflammation, has been associated with atherosclerotic plaques development as well as with destabilization of plaques and promotion of occlusive thrombi.[24] CRP has been shown to injure the glycocalyx of vascular endothelium resulting in dysfunction of endothelium which is considered to be the first step in atherogenesis. The increased levels of CRP have been found in children with OSAS,[25] with actual reduction of these levels after treatment.

Inflammatory Mechanism Causing Neurocognitive Impairment in Obstructive Sleep Apnea Syndrome

Inflammatory pathways were also suggested in the pathophysiology of OSAS-induced cognitive impairment. Gozal and colleagues compared 205 snoring children and 73 non-snoring controls. The snoring children were divided into those with and those without OSAS based on their polysomnographic findings. Both CRP levels and platelet counts were significantly higher in OSAS and more specifically in those with neurocognitive dysfunction.[26]

Inflammatory Markers in Nonobese Children with Obstructive Sleep Apnea Syndrome

Gozal and colleagues followed the levels of IL-6, a pro-inflammatory cytokine, and IL-10, an inhibitor of a broad array of pro-inflammatory immune responses in nonobese children showing increased IL-6 plasma levels and decreased IL-10 plasma levels in children with OSA when compared with healthy children. Furthermore, they have shown that in a substantial proportion of OSA children, treatment with tonsillectomy and adenoidectomy (T&A) will lead to normalization of both IL-6 and IL-10 circulating levels, therefore suggesting inflammatory burden in children with OSAS even without the presence of obesity.[27]

Local Inflammation

Adenotonsillar tissues from children with OSAS were found to have inflammatory cell proliferation and increased expression of pro-inflammatory cytokines and other inflammatory mediators (eg, TNF-a, IL-6, and IL-1a) when compared with adenotonsillar tissues removed from children with recurrent tonsillitis.[28] Studies examining exhaled breath condensate and induced sputum in children with OSAS similarly reveal the upregulation of localized inflammatory processes in upper airway tissues.[29]

Inflammatory Response After Implementation of Obstructive Sleep Apnea Syndrome Treatments

In adult literature CPAP usage in patients with OSA lowered the NF-κB-dependent cytokines TNFα and plasma concentrations of IL-6 and CRP.[30] Similar findings were seen in the pediatric population.

In pediatric patients, Kheirandish-Gozal and colleagues showed that effective treatment of OSA, as evidenced by normalization of respiratory disturbance index during sleep, is associated with prominent improvements in a subset of systemic inflammatory markers, particularly when compared with children in whom AT resulted in less severe, yet clinically significant residual OSA at follow-up.[31,32]

The same group also showed that a 16-week treatment course with montelukast significantly reduces the severity of OSA in children compared with placebo.[33] Assuming that inflammation is the fundamental process leading to OSAS and the use of montelukast assisted with blocking the inflammatory process.

Insomnia and inflammation

Adults with insomnia and objective short sleep duration have been found to be at an increased risk of hypertension, type 2 diabetes, neurocognitive impairment, depression, and mortality.[34] Chronic low-grade inflammation has been proposed as one of the potential paths by which insomnia can lead to adverse health outcomes. Insomnia symptoms and short sleep duration are associated with systemic inflammation in adolescents as well. Few studies looked at short sleep duration in adolescents, as correlated with inflammation. A study in 143 adolescents aged 13 to 18 years found that shorter average sleep duration, as measured by actigraphy, was significantly correlated ($r = 0.29$) with increasing levels of CRP.[35] Fernandez-Mendoza and colleagues looked at 378 adolescents from the Penn State Child Cohort who reported symptoms of insomnia or short sleep time and underwent 9-hour polysomnography followed by a single fasting blood draw to assess plasma levels of CRP and other inflammatory markers. The study showed that elevated CRP levels were primarily present in adolescents who report insomnia symptoms and slept objectively 6 to 7 hour in the laboratory and that this association is independent of demographic factors or comorbid factors frequently associated with insomnia symptoms or inflammation such as depression, anxiety, evening circadian preference, substance use, or medical conditions.

An interesting study by Park and colleagues looked at the pro-inflammatory marker, CRP, in adolescents with inconsistent sleep. The group found correlation between greater weekday/weekend variability and higher CRP. Indicating that altering sleep durations based on the type of days may trigger heightened pro-inflammatory responses during the transition from adolescence to young adulthood.[36]

SUMMARY

There is a bidirectional relationship between sleep and inflammation. Inflammatory cytokines follow a circadian rhythm and the most pronounced are the TNF and IL-6. In return, these cytokines, when excreted during the day in situations of illness or irregular sleep, can cause sleepiness and fatigue. Interrupted sleep, either because of physiologic reasons, such as OSAS, or behavioral causes, such as irregular or short sleep, has cardiovascular, metabolic, and most commonly in pediatrics, cognitive consequences. The line that connects between these sleep consequences is inflammation. In this article, the author discussed the known inflammatory agents that cause the morbidity associated with interrupted sleep, both in the local and systemic level, and showed the mechanisms by which they exert their effect. There has been a significant effort in the past few decades to diagnose and treat sleep-related illnesses, such as OSAS. However, the concept of irregular sleep and short sleep in childhood triggering inflammation and causing equivalent consequences is significant and needs to drive a push for evaluation of normal sleep by pediatricians and other medical providers.

CLINICS CARE POINTS

- Known complications of OSAS, such as neurocognitive dysfunction, cardiovascular morbidities and metabolic complications are likely caused by increase in inflammatory cytokines that mediate the end organ damage. These complications are likely the result of both intermittent hypoxemia and sleep fragmentation. Treatment of OSA decreases the hyper-inflammatory state, as seen by decreased CRP levels.

- Similar increase in inflammation and end organ damage is seen when sleep fragmentation is the only culprit, as seen in individuals with insomnia, short sleep time and irregular sleep pattern.

- Irregular sleep patterns is a modifiable factor that can prevent chronic inflammatory state and its future complications. Review of sleep patterns and intervention when insufficient or irregular sleep is present can have significant impact on the child's future health.

DISCLOSURE

The author has nothing to disclose.

REFERENCE

1. Irwin M. Sleep and inflammation: partners in sickness and in health. Nat Rev Immunol 2019;19(11): 702–15.
2. Krueger JM, Frank MG, Wisor JP, et al. Sleep function: toward elucidating an enigma. Sleep Med Rev 2016;28:46–54.
3. Lange T, Dimitrov S, Born J. Effects of sleep and circadian rhythm on the human immune system. Ann NY Acad Sci 2010;1193:48–59.
4. Vgontzas AN, Papanicolaou DA, Hermida RC, et al. Circadian interleukin-6 secretion and quantity and depth of sleep. J Clin Endocrinol Metab 1999;84: 2603–7.
5. Born J, Lange T, Hansen K, et al. Effects of sleep and circadian rhythm on human circulating immune cells. J Immunol 1997;158:4454–64.
6. Hatipoglu U, Rubinstein I. Inflammation and obstructive sleep apnea syndrome pathogenesis: a Working Hypothesis. Respiration 2003;70:665–71.
7. Vgontzas AN, Papanicolaou DA, Bixler EO. Elevation of plasma cytokines in disorders of excessive daytime sleepiness: role of sleep disturbance and obesity. J Clin Endocrinol Metab 1997;82: 1313–6.
8. Patarca R, Klimas NG, Lutendorf S, et al. Dysregulated expression of tumor necrosis factor in chronic fatigue syndrome: interrelations with cellular sources and patterns of soluble immune mediator expression. Clin Infect Dis 1994;18:S147–53.
9. Visser M, Bouter LM, McQuillan GM, et al. Elevated C-reactive protein levels in overweight and obese adults. JAMA 1999;282:2131–5.
10. Yokoe T, Minoguchi K, Matsuo H, et al. Elevated levels of C-reactive protein and interleukin-6 in

patients with obstructive sleep apnea syndrome are decreased by nasal continuous positive airway pressure. Circulation 2003;107:1129–34.

11. Ip MSM, Lam KSL, Ho C, et al. Serum leptin and vascular risk factors in obstructive sleep apnea. Chest 2000;118:580–6.

12. Tauman R, Ivanenko A, O'Brien LM, et al. Plasma C-reactive protein levels among children with sleep-disordered breathing. Pediatrics 2004; 113(6):e564–9.

13. Kim J, Hakim F, Kheirandish-Gozal L, et al. Inflammatory pathways in children with insufficient or disordered sleep. Respir Physiol Neurobiol 2011; 178(3):465–74.

14. Perkins ND. Integrating cell-signalling pathways with NF-kappaB and IKK function. Nat Rev Mol Cell Biol 2007;8:49–62.

15. Vgontzas AN, Bixler EO, Chrousos GP. Obesity-related sleepiness and fatigue: the role of the stress system and cytokines. Ann N Y Acad Sci 2006;1083: 329–44.

16. Yu YH, Ginsberg HN. Adipocyte signaling and lipid homeostasis: sequelae of insulin-resistant adipose tissue. Circ Res 2005;96:1042–52.

17. Kadowaki T, Yamauchi T. Adiponectin and adiponectin receptors. Endocr Rev 2005;26:439–51.

18. Trzepizur W, Cortese R, Gozal D. Murine models of sleep apnea: functional implications of altered macrophage polarity and epigenetic modifications in adipose and vascular tissues. Metabolism 2018; 84:44–55.

19. Iikuni N, Lam QL, Lu L, et al. Leptin and inflammation. Curr Immunol Rev 2008;4(2):70–9.

20. Lavie L, Lavie P. Molecular mechanisms of cardiovascular disease in OSAHS: the oxidative stress link. Eur Respir J 2009;33(6):1467–84.

21. Gozal D. Sleep, sleep disorders and inflammation in children. Sleep Med 2009;10 1:S12–6.

22. Kritchevsky SB, Cesari M, Pahor M. Inflammatory markers and cardiovascular health in older adults. Cardiovasc Res 2005;66:265–75.

23. Gozal D, Kheirandish-Gozal L, Bhattacharjee R, et al. Neurocognitive and endothelial dysfunction in children with obstructive sleep apnea. Pediatrics 2010;126:e1161–7.

24. Koenig W. High-sensitivity C-reactive protein and atherosclerotic disease: from improved risk prediction to risk-guided therapy. Int J Cardiol 2013; 168(6):5126–34.

25. Li AM, Chan MH, Yin J, et al. C-reactive protein in children with obstructive sleep apnea and the effects of treatment. Pediatr Pulmonol 2008;43(1): 34–40.

26. Gozal D, Crabtree VM, Sans Capdevila O, et al, C-reactive protein, obstructive sleep apnea, and cognitive dysfunction in School-aged children, Am J Respir Crit Care Med 2007;176(2):188–93.

27. Gozal D, Serpero LD, Sans Capdevila O, et al. Systemic inflammation in non-obese children with obstructive sleep apnea. Sleep Med 2008;9(3): 254–9.

28. Kim J, Bhattacharjee R, Dayyat E, et al. Increased cellular proliferation and inflammatory cytokines in tonsils derived from children with obstructive sleep apnea. Pediatr Res 2009;66(4):423–8.

29. Bhattacharjee R, Kim J, Kheirandish-Gozal L, et al. Obesity and obstructive sleep apnea syndrome in children: a tale of inflammatory cascades. Pediatr Pulmonol 2011;46(4):313–23.

30. Bradley TD, Floras JS. Obstructive sleep apnoea and its cardiovascular consequences. Lancet 2009;373(9657):82–93.

31. Kheirandish-Gozal L, Gileles-Hillel A, Alonso-Álvarez ML, et al. Effects of adenotonsillectomy on plasma inflammatory biomarkers in obese children with obstructive sleep apnea: a community-based study. Int J Obes 2015;39(7):1094–100.

32. Kheirandish-Gozal L, Gozal D. Pediatric OSA syndrome morbidity biomarkers. Hunt Is Finally On! CHEST 2017;151(2):500–6.

33. Kheirandish-Gozal L, Bandla HP, Gozal D. Montelukast for children with obstructive sleep apnea: results of a double-blind, randomized, placebo-controlled trial. Ann Am Thorac Soc 2016;13(10): 1736–41.

34. Fernandez-Mendoza J, Baker JH, Alexandros NV, et al. Insomnia symptoms with objective short sleep duration are associated with systemic inflammation in adolescents. Brain Behav Immun 2017;61:110–6.

35. Larkin EK, Rosen CL, Kirschner HL, et al. Variation of C-reactive protein levels in adolescents : association with sleep-disordered breathing and sleep duration. Circulation 2005;111(15):1978–84.

36. Park H, Chiang JJ, Bower JE, et al. Sleep and inflammation during adolescents' transition to young adulthood. J Adolesc Health 2020;67(6):821–8.

Sleep During the Pandemic

Corinne Catarozoli, PhD

KEYWORDS

- Pediatric sleep • COVID-19 pandemic • Sleep disorders

KEY POINTS

- The pandemic significantly disrupted childhood sleep routines, sleep quality, and duration of sleep.
- The increase in mental health issues due to the pandemic exacerbated sleep disturbances.
- Pediatric sleep medicine clinics have adapted practice styles due to pandemic challenges.

BACKGROUND

In March 2020, the World Health Organization (WHO) declared the novel coronavirus outbreak (coronavirus disease 2019 [COVID-19]) to be a global pandemic. The resulting stay-at-home orders and widespread closures disrupted nearly every aspect of family's lives. The COVID-19 pandemic altered daily routines, changed home environments, and increased stress and anxiety. Children and families faced numerous challenges with remote learning, modified parent work schedules, and limited childcare. This abrupt transformation of day-to-day life had a significant impact on many aspects of children's lives including sleep. The manner in which sleep was affected varies across age range but research suggests that infants through adolescents were affected.[1] As the pandemic persists and stretches into a multiple-year period, the nature in which this unprecedented stressor affects families has shifted. This article will review the variety of sleep changes noted at different stages of the pandemic. Contributing factors to these disruptions, including physical activity and outdoor exposure, screen usage, and rising stress and anxiety will be considered. Alterations made by the sleep medicine field to ensure continuity of important sleep services in a safe environment will be discussed, as will areas for future research.

Changes in Childhood Sleep During the Pandemic

During the initial lockdown period in 2020, COVID-19 significantly disrupted day-to-day routines. School, work, and childcare center closures resulted in virtual learning and many parents working remotely from home while simultaneously caring for young children. These modified schedules and arrangements caused numerous changes to family's daily schedules, and as byproduct to sleep, which is highly connected to structure, routine, and predictability. Research on this crisis period has examined the impact of the initial COVID-19 shutdowns on sleep. Dellagiulia and colleagues[2] investigated changes in preschooler sleep during the first 4 weeks of the emergency lockdown in Italy and found that parents reported more challenging bedtime routines and a decrease in child sleep quality. The overall amount of child sleep time decreased initially, then stabilized, suggesting some eventual adjustment. Markovic and colleagues[3] observed a similar pattern of initial disruption followed by a rebound to preconfinement sleep quality with babies and children.

A range of sleep changes has been reported across other studies. Lecuelle and colleagues[4] found that French families with young children aged 6 months to 4 years reported an increase in overall sleep disturbance, decreased number and duration of naps, more difficulty initiating and maintaining sleep, and more frequent parasomnias. Liu and colleagues[5] examined sleep patterns among Chinese preschoolers aged 4 to 6 years and found several distinct differences when compared with a prepandemic sample. Notably, children during the COVID-19 pandemic had later bedtimes and wake times, longer nocturnal but shorter nap duration with comparable overall 24 hours sleep duration. Interestingly,

Department of Psychiatry, Weill Cornell Medicine, 525 East 68th Street, New York, NY 10065, USA
E-mail address: cos2006@med.cornell.edu

Sleep Med Clin 18 (2023) 219–224
https://doi.org/10.1016/j.jsmc.2023.01.004
1556-407X/23/© 2023 Elsevier Inc. All rights reserved.

parents in this study reported fewer sleep disturbances during the pandemic period. Certain behavioral practices were associated with fewer sleep disturbances, including sleeping arrangement (separate rooms or room sharing but not bed sharing), reduced electronic device use, following a regular diet, increased parent–child communication, and harmonious family atmosphere.[5] Room sharing, which increased during the pandemic due to conversion of home space to workspace, is associated with longer sleep onset latency and more parental frustration.[6] Room sharing may also be more likely to occur in low-income families, who were disproportionately affected by the pandemic. Considered together, these studies suggest that changes in children's schedules, even for relatively brief periods, can cause significant disruptions in sleep.

Increased sleep disturbance during the pandemic seems to have affected all ages of younger children[7,8] including infants,[9,10] toddlers,[3,11] and school-age youth.[12–14] Conversely, some studies show that teens and young adults were sleeping more and had fewer sleep issues during the pandemic due to the virtual learning environment.[15] Asynchronous online lessons and elimination of school commutes allow for youth to sleep in later in the morning and may be a more optimal schedule for teenagers. Further, this flexibility may eliminate irregular schedules that typically results from early weekday wakening followed by sleeping in on weekends.[16] In contrast to prepandemic studies that widely demonstrated that teens are sleep-deprived and typically do not receive sufficient hours of overnight sleep, these findings offer a promising upside to virtual learning environments.[17]

Impact of Decreased Activity and Outdoor Exposure on Sleep

Daytime physical activity and daylight exposure have long been linked to positive sleep outcomes for children. During the pandemic, many children were faced with staying indoors all day resulting in less sunlight exposure and physical activity. Particularly for families who did not have access to outdoor space within their home, children had more sedentary time than typical. Shinomiya and colleagues[10] found that parents reported decreased outdoor play for both babies and toddlers. A global study of 3-to-5-year-old children during the pandemic showed that children had more sedentary screen time, decreased outdoor time, and worse sleep habits.[18] Children who could go outside were more likely to meet WHO movement guidelines and parents whose children

sleep worsened during the pandemic attributed reduced exercise as a factor in this exacerbation.[19] In a study of Canadian children during the pandemic, only as minority (18%) met physical activity recommendations,[20] and this percentage continued to worsen during subsequent waves of the virus.[21] These findings all continue to point to physical activity and outdoor time as important contributors to healthy sleep habits in children.

Impact of Stress and Anxiety on Sleep

The pandemic has clearly brought with it enormous amounts of stress for children and families because they navigated an unknown virus, disruptive school closures, balancing working from home with childcare, and increased isolation. Rates of mental health issues, particularly anxiety and depression, have drastically increased among youth during the pandemic.[22,23] In 2021, the US Surgeon General issued an advisory warning of the unprecedented levels of mental health disorders since the start of the pandemic, including a doubling of anxiety and depression symptoms and increasing rates of ER visits for suicidality.[24] The American Academy of Pediatrics (AAP), American Academy of Child and Adolescent Psychiatry, and Children's Hospital Association similarly issued a declaration of a national emergency in child and adolescent mental health driven by the stress of the pandemic.

Pervasive anxiety and worry about virus exposure, loss of loved ones, missed milestones, and social isolation have marked the experience of many adolescents during the pandemic. Teens have witnessed parents who are stressed by job instability, financial concerns, and food insecurity. Stress has long been linked with poor sleep quality and duration, and sleep disturbances are hallmark symptoms of anxiety and depression. Thus, with growing rates of mental illness, come increasing sleep issues among youth. Research during the pandemic has shown that anxiety symptoms in youth are linked with sleep disturbance.[25]

Parental mental health has also been linked to childhood sleep disturbance during the pandemic. Top and Cam found that youth of parents who felt helpless, apprehensive, and frightened during the pandemic experienced more sleep difficulties.[14] Similarly, children of mothers with acute levels of anxiety had worse sleep quality.[26] Caregiver stress level has been identified as an important risk factor for lower sleep quality in both babies and young children.[3] A study examining sleep quality in children who were medically hospitalized during COVID-19 found that they had worse sleep, despite having fewer overnight room entries, which historically are associated with reduced sleep quality. Caregivers attributed the poor sleep quality to increased stress and anxiety, and parents themselves also expressed feeling more sad, weary, and less calm during this time as compared with prepandemic.[27] The record levels of mental health issues facing youth and parents today are yet another pandemic byproduct that will need to be addressed going forward.

Impact of Screen Use on Sleep

Excessive screen time has long been established as detrimental to sleep for a variety of reasons. Exposure to bright light and the subsequent impact on melatonin production, engagement in potentially arousing or stressful activities, and the displacement of sleep-inducing activities such as exercise are all potential contributors to this relationship. Using screens in bed can be particularly problematic for sleep initiation, and the AAP recommends youth avoid screens for at least 1 hour before bedtime. With the transition to virtual learning and lack of available alternative activities, although, youth have been spending increased amounts of time on electronics during the pandemic.[28,29] Although some increase was inevitable as virtual school was the primary learning modality for most children, screen time use has extended beyond educational purposes, and many youth report using electronics for social media, texting, video chatting, streaming services, video games, and Internet browsing during lockdown.[29] Bruni and colleagues[15] found that school-age children increased screen time to 3 to 4 h/d, excluding school lessons. Even parents of infants reported longer television and smartphone use times for their babies.[10] Notably, more screen use was associated with poorer mental health and greater perceived stress, as well as sleep disturbance.[25,29]

Sleep Recommendations During a Pandemic

The Society of Behavioral Sleep Medicine convened a COVID-19 task force to address worsening sleep issues during the pandemic and offer guidance for providers. The task force suggested that attaining healthy sleep during a crisis period such as the pandemic may be supported by optimizing sleep schedules, limiting sleep-interfering factors, and increasing routine daytime behavior.[30] Maintaining a consistent routine with regular wake times, mealtimes, activity times, and bedtime is crucial to support children's sleep. Parents can help children manage anxiety at bedtime through the practice of relaxation techniques (ie, diaphragmatic breathing, progressive muscle relaxation, guided imagery). Families should maintain prepandemic sleeping arrangements, to the extent possible, and encourage children to fall asleep independently without the presence of a parent. Behavioral interventions such as reward systems and gradual withdrawal of parents for difficult bedtime behavior remain very relevant. Limiting electronics use (tablet, television, smartphone) for at least an hour before bedtime and leaving devices outside the bedroom is particularly pertinent during a time of such increased screen time.

Changes to Pediatric Sleep Medicine Practice

The onset of the COVID-19 pandemic led to an abrupt halt of most in-person pediatric sleep medicine services. Many sleep centers were forced to temporarily close office and laboratory space due to stay-at-home orders and discontinuation of nonessential services across most medical center or practices.[31] For a period of time, overnight sleep studies, pulmonary function test (PFT) laboratories, and surgical procedures related to sleep disturbances were unavailable. Even as the initial crisis period of COVID-19 has waned, ongoing social distancing requirements make traditional sleep medicine practices difficult to operate. These challenges necessitated a quick and creative rethinking of delivering sleep medicine services for children to ensure continuity of care.

Although home sleep apnea tests (HSATs) are not recommended for pediatric patients by the American Academy of Sleep Medicine,[32] some sleep centers relied on these as an alternative option when in-person studies were available during the height of the pandemic.[33,34] Going forward, HSATs may reasonably be considered for postpubertal teenagers or children with developmental delays, for whom the sleep laboratory environment is difficult to tolerate.[34] As the initial COVID-19 surge declined, sleep and PFT laboratories, as well as nonessential surgical procedures have largely resumed with new guidelines around safety, screening, and personal protective equipment.

Telemedicine has effectively been leveraged to allow for safe continuation of many sleep services during the ongoing pandemic period.[35] Behavioral sleep medicine is particularly well suited to telemedicine because these visits do not involve any physical examination, obtaining vitals, or other procedures requiring a patient to be physically present.[36] Particularly for parents of babies or toddlers, where recommendations are parent-directed, virtual visits allow for them to be seen at a convenient time without children present, which may allow for better uptake of information.[33] Research suggests that the efficacy of many sleep interventions is not diminished through the virtual format. Cognitive behavioral therapy for insomnia, for instance, has been shown to be effective when delivered via the Internet.[37] CPAP follow-up has also been identified as ideal for telemedicine.[38]

Telemedicine has added benefits of reducing school and work absences, having multiple caregivers present at once, reducing time, travel, and clinic space costs, and increased efficiency for providers.[39] Multidisciplinary approaches to sleep medicine with a variety of providers (pulmonology, psychology, neurology) can easily and efficiently see patients together in one virtual appointment while not being physically present in the same location. Many of these virtual services will likely continue on postpandemic due to convenience and patient preference.

Sleep Medicine Training

The temporary halt of sleep services posed a concern for fewer clinical training opportunities available in medical or psychology education programs. Given the profound impact the pandemic has had on pediatric sleep, the demand for these services has increased, and the field needs competent providers to sustain a workforce to meet this need. Fortunately, the pivot to telemedicine now introduces a new opportunity for trainees to observe and participate in sleep-related care. Leveraging technology for didactics and teaching also provides new and exciting opportunities for this generation of trainees.[36]

Future Research Considerations

Pediatric sleep researchers rapidly mobilized to study the impact of the pandemic on sleep through a variety of cross-sectional and retrospective designs.[40] Longitudinal data are more limited, and implementing interventional or experimental studies has been difficult due to numerous barriers. Ongoing gaps in the literature include how the COVID-19 virus itself affects childhood sleep, both in the short-term and in relation to "long-COVID," as well as the effect of the pandemic on children with premorbid primary sleep disorders.[40] Studying the efficacy of telemedicine sleep services continues to be important as the virtual format remains a primary delivery mode.

SUMMARY

In sum, the COVID-19 pandemic significantly affected childhood sleep. Early confinement periods led to more challenging bedtime routines and a decrease in child sleep quality. Decreased outdoor time, daylight exposure, and physical activity levels, and huge increases in screen time have likely further contributed to these disruptions. Although some of these sleep problems may have stabilized once the initial lockdown periods abated, other sleep-related challenges have persisted as the pandemic continues. The mental health crisis remains a substantial threat to positive sleep outcomes as raising anxiety and depression rates overwhelm today's youth. Tied to this, parental mental health, which is related to child sleep quality, is being significantly taxed.

To support ongoing sleep issues among youth, sleep medicine practices have had to adapt and evolve during the COVID-19 pandemic. An urgent shutdown of nonessential sleep services led to a quick and robust growth of telemedicine. Although most in-person sleep studies, PFT laboratories, and surgical procedures have resumed with additional safety precautions in place, telemedicine will likely remain a primary delivery modality for sleep services given the many benefits. Adaptations for sleep medicine training and research in the face of pandemic challenges should also be considered.

CLINICS CARE POINTS

- During the initial lockdown period of the pandemic, children experienced increased sleep disturbances including later bedtimes, decreased number and duration of naps, more difficulty initiating and maintaining sleep, and more frequent parasomnias
- Decreased outdoor time and daylight exposure along with increased sedentary behavior during the pandemic have contributed to childhood sleep problems
- The transition to virtual learning and general increases in screen use contributed to sleep disturbances among adolescents
- Significant increases in anxiety, depression, and other mental health symptoms during the pandemic are linked to sleep difficulties
- Pediatric sleep centers were faced with an abrupt halt to in-person services such as sleep studies, PFT laboratories, and surgical procedures
- Telemedicine has effectively been implemented to offer many sleep services remotely

DECLARATION OF INTERESTS

The author has nothing to disclose.

REFERENCES

1. Stearns MA, Ievers-Landis CE, McCrae CS, et al. Sleep across childhood during the COVID-19 pandemic: a narrative review of the literature and clinical case examples. Child Health Care 2022; 51(4):408–30.
2. Dellagiulia A, Lionetti F, Fasolo M, et al. Early impact of COVID-19 lockdown on children's sleep: a 4-week longitudinal study. J Clin Sleep Med 2020;16(9): 1639–40.
3. Markovic A, Mühlematter C, Beaugrand M, et al. Severe effects of the COVID-19 confinement on young children's sleep: a longitudinal study identifying risk and protective factors. J Sleep Res 2021;30(5): e13314.
4. Lecuelle F, Leslie W, Huguelet S, et al. Did the COVID-19 lockdown really have no impact on young children's sleep? J Clin Sleep Med 2020;16(12): 2121.
5. Liu Z, Tang H, Jin Q, et al. Sleep of preschoolers during the coronavirus disease 2019 (COVID-19) outbreak. J Sleep Res 2021;30(1):e13142.
6. Gupta G, O'Brien LM, Dang LT, et al. Sleep of infants and toddlers during 12 months of the COVID-19 pandemic in the midwestern United States. J Clin Sleep Med 2022;18(5):1225–34.
7. Bacaro V, Chiabudini M, Buonanno C, et al. Sleep characteristics in Italian children during home confinement due to COVID-19 outbreak. Clinical Neuropsychiatry 2021;18(1):13.
8. Sharma M, Aggarwal S, Madaan P, et al. Impact of COVID-19 pandemic on sleep in children and adolescents: a systematic review and meta-analysis. Sleep Med 2021;84:259–67.
9. Kahn M, Barnett N, Glazer A, et al. Infant sleep during COVID-19: longitudinal analysis of infants of US mothers in home confinement versus working as usual. Sleep Health 2021;7(1):19–23.
10. Shinomiya Y, Yoshizaki A, Murata E, et al. Sleep and the general behavior of infants and parents during the closure of schools as a result of the COVID-19 Pandemic: comparison with 2019 data. Children 2021;8(2):168.
11. Di Giorgio E, Di Riso D, Mioni G, et al. The interplay between mothers' and children behavioral and psychological factors during COVID-19: an Italian study. Eur Child Adolesc Psychiatry 2021;30(9): 1401–12.
12. Cellini N, Di Giorgio E, Mioni G, et al. Sleep and psychological difficulties in Italian school-age children during COVID-19 lockdown. J Pediatr Psychol 2021;46(2):153–67.
13. Luma N.B., Sleep patterns and sleep disturbance in school-age children amid COVID-19 pandemic outbreak, European J Psychological Research, 9 (1), 2022, 1-10.
14. Top FU, Cam HH. Sleep disturbances in school-aged children 6–12 years during the COVID-19 pandemic in Turkey. J Pediatr Nurs 2022;63:125–30.
15. Bruni O, Malorgio E, Doria M, et al. Changes in sleep patterns and disturbances in children and adolescents in Italy during the Covid-19 outbreak. Sleep Med 2022;91:166–74.
16. Wright KP Jr, Linton SK, Withrow D, et al. Sleep in university students prior to and during COVID-19 Stay-at-Home orders. Curr Biol 2020;30(14):R797–8.
17. Yuen K, Strang AR, Flynn-Evans EE, et al. Child and teen sleep and pandemic-era school. J Clin Sleep Med 2021;17(4):613–5.
18. Okely AD, Kariippanon KE, Guan H, et al. Global effect of COVID-19 pandemic on physical activity, sedentary behaviour and sleep among 3-to 5-year-old children: a longitudinal study of 14 countries. BMC Public Health 2021;21(1):1–15.
19. MacKenzie NE, Keys E, Hall WA, et al. Children's sleep during COVID-19: how sleep influences surviving and thriving in families. J Pediatr Psychol 2021;46(9):1051–62.
20. Guerrero MD, Vanderloo LM, Rhodes RE, et al. Canadian children's and youth's adherence to the 24-h movement guidelines during the COVID-19 pandemic: a decision tree analysis. Journal of Sport and Health Science 2020;9(4):313–21.
21. Moore SA, Faulkner G, Rhodes RE, et al. Few Canadian children and youth were meeting the 24-hour movement behaviour guidelines 6-months into the COVID-19 pandemic: follow-up from a national study. Appl Physiol Nutr Metabol 2021;46(10): 1225–40.
22. Racine N, McArthur BA, Cooke JE, et al. Global prevalence of depressive and anxiety symptoms in children and adolescents during COVID-19: a meta-analysis. JAMA Pediatr 2021;175(11): 1142–50.
23. Ma L, Mazidi M, Li K, et al. Prevalence of mental health problems among children and adolescents during the COVID-19 pandemic: a systematic review and meta-analysis. J Affect Disord 2021;293:78–89.
24. Office of the Surgeon General (OSG). Protecting youth mental health: the U.S. Surgeon General's Advisory. Washington (DC): US Department of Health and Human Services; 2021.
25. Refay E, Sayed A, Hashem SA, et al. Sleep quality and anxiety symptoms in Egyptian children and adolescents during COVID-19 pandemic lockdown. Bull Natl Res Cent 2021;45(1):1–8.
26. Zreik G, Asraf K, Haimov I, et al. Maternal perceptions of sleep problems among children and mothers during the coronavirus disease 2019 (COVID-19) pandemic in Israel. J Sleep Res 2021; 30(1):e13201.
27. Riehm JM, Arora VM, Tatineni S, et al. The impact of the COVID-19 pandemic on nighttime room entries

and sleep disruptions for pediatric patients. Sleep Med 2021;84:76–81.

28. Moraleda-Cibrián M, Albares-Tendero J, Pin-Arboledas G. Screen media use and sleep patterns in Spanish adolescents during the lockdown of the coronavirus pandemic. Sleep Breath 2022;26:1–8.

29. Nagata JM, Magid HSA, Gabriel KP. Screen time for children and adolescents during the coronavirus disease 2019 pandemic. Obesity 2020;28(9):1582–3.

30. Crew EC, Baron KG, Grandner MA, et al. The society of behavioral sleep medicine (SBSM) COVID-19 task force: objectives and summary recommendations for managing sleep during a pandemic. Behav Sleep Med 2020;18(4):570–2.

31. Johnson KG, Sullivan SS, Nti A, et al. The impact of the COVID-19 pandemic on sleep medicine practices. J Clin Sleep Med 2021;17(1):79–87.

32. Kirk V, Baughn J, D'Andrea L, et al. American Academy of Sleep Medicine position paper for the use of a home sleep apnea test for the diagnosis of OSA in children. J Clin Sleep Med 2017;13(10):1199–203.

33. Donskoy I, Loghmanee D, Fields BG, et al. Telemedicine-based sleep services for a complex child: optimizing care during a pandemic and beyond. J Clin Sleep Med 2022;18(1):325–7.

34. Sullivan S, Anastasi M, Beam E, et al. Opportunities and unknowns in adapting pediatric sleep practices

to a pandemic world. J Clin Sleep Med 2021;17(3):361–2.

35. Taylor JB, Oermann CM, Deterding RR, et al. Innovating and adapting in pediatric pulmonology and sleep medicine during the COVID-19 pandemic: ATS pediatric assembly web committee consensus statement for initial COVID-19 virtual response. Pediatr Pulmonol 2021;56(2):539–50.

36. Owens J, Katwa U, Sheldon S, et al. Uncharted territory: challenges and opportunities in pediatric sleep medicine during the COVID-19 pandemic and beyond part I: clinical services and teaching and training issues. Sleep Med 2021;88:285.

37. De Bruin EJ, Bögels SM, Oort FJ, et al. Improvements of adolescent psychopathology after insomnia treatment: results from a randomized controlled trial over 1 year. JCPP (J Child Psychol Psychiatry) 2018;59(5):509–22.

38. Katwa U, Owens J, Sheldon S, et al. Uncharted territory: challenges and opportunities in pediatric sleep medicine during the COVID-19 pandemic and beyond part II: the sleep laboratory. Sleep Med 2021;88:282–4.

39. Paruthi S. Telemedicine in pediatric sleep. Sleep Med Clin 2020;15(3):e1–7.

40. Gruber R. Challenges and opportunities related to pediatric sleep research during the Covid-19 pandemic. Sleep 2021;44(12):zsab255.

Health Disparities in Pediatric Sleep

Francesca Lupini, MS[a], Ariel A. Williamson, PhD, DBSM[b,c],*

KEYWORDS

- Adolescence • Disparities • Early childhood • Health equity • Middle childhood • Pediatrics • Sleep

KEY POINTS

- Cross-sectional and longitudinal research has established that there are disparities in pediatric sleep health and sleep disorders by race, ethnicity, and socioeconomic status from birth through adolescence.
- Factors at multiple socioecological levels (ie, child, family, school, health-care system, neighborhood, and sociocultural), including historical and ongoing racism, discrimination, and oppression, contribute to these disparities.
- Mechanistic research and studies using an intersectional lens to understand overlapping marginalized identities are needed to advance sleep health disparities research.
- Interventions addressing multilevel socioecological determinants of disparities are needed to promote pediatric sleep health equity.

PEDIATRIC SLEEP HEALTH DISPARITIES

The National Institute of Minority Health and Health Disparities (NIMHD) defines a health disparity as a health difference that adversely affects disadvantaged populations on one or more health outcomes.[1] Health disparity populations include individuals from racially and ethnically minoritized backgrounds, those of lower socioeconomic status (SES) backgrounds, gender minorities, rural populations, and those with identities at the intersection of these and other categories. This article reviews disparities in pediatric sleep health and sleep disorders and potential determinants of these disparities. Much of this research focuses on disparities by race and ethnicity, which are sociopolitical constructs.[2,3] Observed disparities do not result from biological differences by race and ethnicity but rather are a manifestation of historical and ongoing racism, discrimination, and oppression that produce differential exposure to adverse social and environmental factors. Accordingly, we apply a socioecological framework[4] to examine interacting social and environmental factors that may contribute to pediatric sleep health disparities and their related outcomes (**Fig. 1**). These factors exist at multiple levels of the social ecology, including the individual child and family levels, the educational and health-care systems levels, and the broader neighborhood/community level and sociocultural context.

As defined by Buysse[5] and expanded for pediatrics,[6] sleep health is a multidimensional construct that encompasses sleep patterns (eg, duration, continuity/awakenings), perceived sleep quality, alertness, and sleep-related behaviors (eg, bedtime routines, electronics usage). Sleep disorders in this review include behavioral concerns, such as insomnia and related symptoms (eg, broad caregiver-perceived or child/adolescent-perceived sleep problems, difficulty falling/returning to sleep) and medically based concerns.[7]

[a] Children's National Hospital, 111 Michigan Avenue Northwest, 6 Floor CTR Suite, Room M7658, Washington, DC 20010, USA; [b] Children's Hospital of Philadelphia, Roberts Center for Pediatric Research, 2716 South Street Boulevard, Room 8202, Philadelphia, PA 19146, USA; [c] University of Pennsylvania, Perelman School of Medicine, Philadelphia, PA 19104, USA
* Corresponding author. Children's Hospital of Philadelphia, Roberts Center for Pediatric Research, 2716 South Street Boulevard, Room 8202, Philadelphia, PA 19146.
E-mail address: williamsoa@chop.edu

Sleep Med Clin 18 (2023) 225–234
https://doi.org/10.1016/j.jsmc.2023.01.005
1556-407X/23/© 2023 Elsevier Inc. All rights reserved.

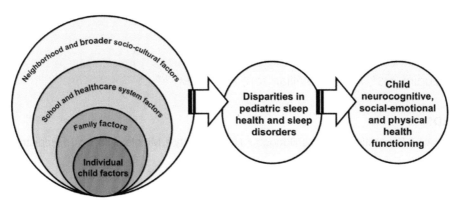

Fig. 1. Socioecological framework applied to determinants and consequences of pediatric sleep health disparities.

Sleep disorder disparities research is mostly limited to insomnia and sleep disordered breathing (SDB). We review racial, ethnic, and socioeconomic disparities in sleep health and these sleep disorders by age, from early childhood (ages 0–5 years) through middle childhood (6–11 years) and adolescence (12–18 years). We then discuss socioecological contributors to these disparities and future research directions.

DISPARITIES IN SLEEP HEALTH
Early Childhood

Research primarily conducted in the United States (US) has demonstrated that racial, ethnic, and socioeconomic sleep health disparities begin in early development. Most studies have examined sleep duration, continuity (awakenings), and behaviors, particularly bedtime routines. Studies of infants and toddlers show that those of African American/Black (hereafter, "Black"), Hispanic/Latinx (hereafter, "Latinx"), and Asian backgrounds tend to obtain less sleep than their non-Hispanic/Latinx White (hereafter, "White") counterparts.[8–13] A study following 194 infants from ages 1 to 6 months found that Latinx infants' nighttime sleep duration was approximately 30 minutes less at 1 month and an hour less at 6 months compared with White infants.[9] These racial differences in nighttime sleep duration have persisted during the coronavirus pandemic.[10] A systematic review of sleep in 2 to 5 year olds found that White children had longer nighttime sleep duration and napped less frequently than Black and Latinx children,[14] suggesting that disparities in nighttime sleep duration could be due to differences in daytime sleep. Nonetheless, longitudinal research has demonstrated that despite differences in napping, total (24 hours) sleep duration was shorter in Black, Latinx, and Asian infants from birth to age 2, by approximately 24 minutes, 49 minutes, and 57 fewer minutes of sleep per day, respectively, compared with White infants.[11]

In some studies, when adjusting for family SES, racial, and ethnic differences in sleep duration attenuate for Latinx and Black children but remain or become stronger for Asian children.[12,15] A study of 9-month-olds modeled cumulative exposure to multiple family SES variables, such as maternal education and family poverty, and found that greater cumulative risks were associated with a long sleep onset latency and/or frequent and long night awakenings.[16] There is also evidence that young children living in lower-SES neighborhoods, typically indexed according to US Census data, experience later bedtimes, a long sleep onset latency, and short sleep duration compared with those in higher SES neighborhoods, although this research does not always include both family and neighborhood SES.[17,18] A study of 80 Black infants found that after controlling for family SES, infants in lower-SES neighborhoods had more night awakenings, suggesting unique neighborhood-level links with sleep.[19]

Most early childhood sleep health research has focused on bedtime routines, with a systematic review showing that consistent bedtime routines are less prevalent among Latinx and Black children compared with White children.[14] In addition to this finding, a study of 3217 3-year-olds found that children with a mother who had less education, those with a lower family income, and those in larger households were also less likely to have a bedtime routine.[20] In another study, greater cumulative risk, indexed by family and neighborhood SES as well as caregiver depressive symptoms, was associated with greater likelihood of poor sleep health, including an inconsistent bedtime routine, insufficient sleep duration, and caffeine consumption.[21]

Middle Childhood

A systematic review of racial and ethnic sleep health disparities in children aged 6 to 19 years found that across ages, White youth consistently obtain more sleep than Black and Latinx youth, with inconclusive results for Asian youth.[22] A study of 1293 youth aged 6 to 12 years found that Asian, Black, and Latinx children slept an average of 23, 17, and 14 minutes less than White children.[23] A previously discussed longitudinal study found that at every time point from birth to age 7, Black, Latinx, and Asian children were more likely to obtain insufficient sleep compared with White children, although including SES in analyses attenuated differences for Black and Latinx children.[12]

Compared with early childhood research, fewer studies of socioeconomic sleep health disparities have been conducted with school-aged children. In a study of socioeconomic position (SEP), objective SEP (family income) was related to self-reported child sleep duration, whereas subjective SEP was related to daytime sleepiness and caregiver-reported sleep duration but only in children aged 8 to 13 years but not adolescents.[24] In another study, children who grew up in neighborhoods with historically high poverty were more likely to exhibit insufficient sleep duration.[25] A study of third-grade and fourth-grade children examined associations among multiple SES indicators and actigraphic sleep, and moderation by race and ethnicity.[26] Poor caregiver-perceived economic well-being was linked to short actigraphy-derived sleep minutes and variable sleep onset, while children attending impoverished schools had a short sleep duration. Lower maternal education was linked to low sleep efficiency in Black but not White children, underscoring the importance of examining race, ethnicity, and multiple SES indicators.

Adolescence

As in research on school-aged children, most adolescent sleep health disparities studies have focused on sleep duration. In a systematic review, Black youth obtained less sleep than White and Latinx youth but findings for Asian youth were inconclusive.[22] A study of 1543 adolescents found that Black and Latinx youth reported shorter sleep duration than both White and Asian youth.[27] The same study found race by gender interactions, with Latinx men obtaining less sleep than White and Asian men, and Black women obtaining less sleep than White women. Another study found that Black adolescents obtained approximately 35 minutes less sleep and more actigraphy-derived wake after sleep onset than both Latinx and Asian youth.[28] Another study has shown short

actigraphy-derived nighttime sleep duration[29] and fragmented sleep[30] in Black versus White adolescents, although in one study total 24-hour sleep duration did not differ by race.[29]

With regard to socioeconomic disparities, a study of adolescents found that those of lower SES backgrounds had a longer sleep onset, shorter duration, and greater weekday to weeknight variability compared with youth of higher-SES.[31] In another study of multiple objective and subjective SES factors, objective SEP was related to adolescents' perceived sleep disturbances, whereas subjective SEP was associated with poor self-reported sleep quality and short caregiver-reported child sleep duration.[24] Lower SES may also exacerbate linkages between poor sleep health and adolescent functioning.[32] Adjusting for race and ethnicity, shorter and less efficient actigraphy-derived sleep patterns in older adolescents were linked to worse cognitive and behavioral functioning but only among youth from lower SES backgrounds.[32]

BEHAVIORAL SLEEP DISPARITIES
Early Childhood

One of the few studies examining racial and ethnic differences in caregiver-perceived child sleep problems found that a higher proportion of White mothers of preschoolers reported concerns about their child's difficulty falling asleep compared with Black but not Latina mothers.[33] In another study, Black caregivers reported increased preschooler bedtime difficulties compared with White caregivers but there were no racial differences in the proportion of caregiver-reported overall child sleep problems.[34] A study of sleep disorders diagnosed in primary care found that White infants and toddlers were more likely to receive any sleep disorder diagnosis, including insomnia, than those from Black or "other" racial and ethnic backgrounds.[7] With regard to socioeconomic variation, research on 14,980 young children found that caregivers living in neighborhoods with the lowest SES, determined via a US Census-based index, were less likely to report a child sleep problem than those in higher SES neighborhoods, despite shorter caregiver-reported child sleep duration and longer sleep onset latencies among those in lower SES neighborhoods.[18] Research also indicates that preschoolers exposed to greater cumulative risks, including lower family and neighborhood SES, were more likely to have caregiver-reported insomnia symptoms.[21]

Middle Childhood

Some school-based research suggests increased caregiver-reported child sleep problems in Latinx and Black children (94%) compared with a sample of predominantly White children (23%).[35,36] A retrospective study found that White patients were more likely than Black patients to present to a pediatric sleep clinic with behavioral sleep problems, such as difficulty falling asleep, than with medically-based sleep concerns.[37] A study of 271 children showed that having a lower SES background was associated with increased perceived sleep/wake problems and greater daytime sleepiness.[38] Other studies have examined interrelations among sociodemographic factors, sleep, and child outcomes. For instance, Black children with sleep problems had worse cognitive and academic functioning compared with White children with sleep problems.[39] In another study, Black children experiencing financial hardship exhibited a more variable sleep onset and more self-reported sleep problems compared with Black children without financial hardship, while no such pattern occurred in White children.[26]

Adolescence

Longitudinal research on a large cohort of youth with childhood insomnia symptoms (CISs) has demonstrated that symptoms tend to persist in Black and Latinx compared with White adolescents.[40] CIS persistence rates were higher in White youth from lower SES backgrounds compared with White youth from higher SES backgrounds, whereas persistence rates were higher in racially and ethnically minoritized youth regardless of SES. Trouble sleeping in older adolescents, which may reflect insomnia or the circadian disturbances that are prevalent among teenagers, also varies by family and neighborhood SES. Among older adolescents, lower perceived neighborhood cohesion was associated with trouble sleeping, and this effect was stronger in adolescents with lower maternal education.[41] One study found that Latinx adolescents reported fewer difficulties maintaining sleep than non-Latinx adolescents,[42] whereas another study found no differences among Black, Latinx, and White adolescents in insomnia prevalence.[43] In a study of multiple sociodemographic factors, adolescents identifying as "Mexican" (vs "Mexican-American") and foreign-born youth were at lower risk for insomnia, and those from lower SES backgrounds were higher risk for insomnia.[44]

MEDICAL SLEEP DISPARITIES
Early Childhood

Few studies have examined early childhood disparities in medical sleep disorders. Research is generally limited to SDB, a spectrum of breathing difficulties during sleep from mild snoring to severe obstructive sleep apnea (OSA).[45,46] One study found that Black infants and toddlers (25%) were more likely to exhibit habitual snoring ($\geq$3 nights/wk) than White children (15%).[47] In another study, Black and Latinx preschoolers were more than twice as likely than White children to have SDB symptoms.[48] A Canadian study found that children aged 2 to 8 years with OSA were more likely to reside in more densely populated neighborhoods with lower average rates of family income and more single-parent households.[49]

Middle Childhood and Adolescence

SDB affects approximately 10% to 17% of children, with 1% to 3% experiencing OSA.[50,51] Black youth are 4 to 6 times more likely to experience SDB than White youth,[46,52] with some evidence of increased OSA severity on polysomnogram in Black compared with White children.[53] Children from lower-SES families and neighborhoods are also more likely to experience SDB than those living in higher SES contexts.[54–56] Disparities also exist in SDB treatment, likely due to differential access to and contact with the health-care system. Several studies indicate that OSA treatment via adenotonsillectomy is less prevalent in Black and Latinx compared with White youth.[54,57–59] A recent study found that Black and Latinx youth with Medicaid insurance were less likely to receive SDB surgical treatment compared with White youth, who also had shorter wait times for surgery.[60] Some research suggests that adenotonsillectomy for OSA may not improve OSA-related behavioral symptoms as much in Black youth compared with those of White and other racial and ethnic backgrounds.[59] Studies using insurance as a proxy for SES have additionally found that compared with those with private insurance, publicly insured youth tend to have lower adenotonsillectomy rates and greater SDB treatment delays, both in initial polysomnography and surgeries.[57,61]

MULTILEVEL DETERMINANTS OF PEDIATRIC SLEEP DISPARITIES

Bronfenbrenner's socioecological framework[4] (see **Fig. 1**) has been applied to understand contributors to pediatric sleep health[6] and to sleep health disparities across the life span[62] and in pediatric SDB.[63] The factors outlined below are not an exhaustive list of contributors. Future research is needed to identify how these, and other modifiable factors, can be leveraged to promote sleep health equity. Given its multilevel nature, racism (eg, systemic, structural, institutional; personally mediated; and internalized)[64–67] and discrimination are included at each socioecological level.

Child Level

Child characteristics such as prematurity, respiratory issues, and obesity are linked with variation in sleep patterns and SDB and may contribute to disparities.[46,52] Early childhood temperament may also influence sleep patterns as a function of caregiver characteristics, such as mood or parenting style.[68,69] For example, compared with infants with "easy" temperaments, those with "difficult" temperaments exhibit poor sleep outcomes, including frequent night awakenings and short sleep duration.[69] A longitudinal study following mother–infant dyads from birth to age 6 months found that infant temperament moderated maternal emotional availability at bedtime and infant sleep duration, with high-surgency infants exhibiting greater increases in sleep duration in the context of higher maternal bedtime emotional availability.[70] As parenting behaviors vary cross-culturally, more research is needed on these linkages in racially and ethnically minoritized families and in other countries/regions.

Personally mediated and/or internalized racism and discrimination are other child-level factors linked with poor sleep, primarily in adolescents.[28,71–73] Daily discrimination was related to increased same-night sleep disturbances and next-day sleepiness in Asian, Black, and Latinx teens,[28] which could contribute to racial and ethnic sleep health disparities. A study of college students also found that discrimination was related to poor sleep, and that this association was stronger among students who also reported higher levels of internalized racism.[71]

Family Level

Sleep health literacy and beliefs are family factors that also may contribute to sleep health disparities. Lower sleep health literacy, which is correlated with SES, has been associated with poor child sleep health.[74,75] Research also shows that the negative sleep-related impacts of having a television in the bedroom are more pronounced among racially and ethnically minoritized children compared with their White peers.[76] Qualitative research indicates that limited sleep health knowledge may contribute to poor sleep in racially and ethnically minoritized adolescents.[77,78] One of these studies was conducted with American Indian/Alaska Native (AI/AN) teens, who described the importance of family cohesion in helping to maintain stable sleep environments and, in turn, optimal sleep health.[77]

The sleep environment, which includes sleep arrangements (ie, bed-sharing and room-sharing) as well as light, noise, and temperature, among other factors,[79] likely contributes to sleep health disparities. Families of lower-SES may need to bed-share and/or room-share due to limited resources, whereas other families may practice bed-sharing intentionally, as part of their cultural practices and/or preferences, or in response to a child sleep problem.[80,81] Generally, African and Asian countries/regions exhibit higher rates of bed-sharing compared with European and American countries/regions.[80,82] In one US study of families from low-SES backgrounds, Black and Latinx families were more likely to bed-share than White families.[83] The effects of sleep arrangements on child sleep are mixed, and likely depend on the context in which families are bed-sharing/room-sharing. Understanding this context is crucial for identifying how sleep arrangements and aspects of the sleep environment can be enhanced to promote sleep health equity, particularly among families experiencing noisy, crowded, and/or transitional sleep environments.

Qualitative research has also revealed that caregivers cite family work/school schedules, household responsibilities, and other family members' sleep schedules as barriers to child and family sleep health.[84–86] Among Black adolescents, more household chaos was associated with greater disruptions to youth sleep by other household members' behaviors, including electronics use and evening social visits.[87] Family irregularity has been longitudinally associated with more reported child sleep problems, short sleep duration, and long sleep onset.[88] Household chaos and family relationships are associated with child sleep in several other studies.[89] For instance, there is evidence that household chaos mediates associations between positive parenting and sleep health, and between family resources and child sleep duration.[90,91] One study found that better parent–child relationships were associated with decreased insomnia risk, particularly among Latinx adolescents compared with White and Black youth.[92]

Family members' experiences of racism and discrimination are also linked to child sleep. Caregiver experiences of racial discrimination, for example, are associated with short early childhood sleep duration.[93] Caregivers' experiences of racism may also impact factors associated with child sleep, including caregiver mood,[64–66] parenting,[67] and caregivers' own sleep.[94] A study of gendered racial discrimination found that higher levels of mothers' gendered racial stress was directly associated with poor child sleep, although racial/ethnic discrimination was not.[95] This finding highlights the importance of intersectionality in research on the role of racism and discrimination in sleep health disparities.

School/Health-Care Level

Although racism at the school and health-care system levels has not been studied in relation to child sleep, biases in these systems likely contribute to disparities in sleep-related outcomes and treatments. Research shows that teachers and health-care providers hold implicit pro-White/anti-Black biases, which can affect teacher–student and provider–patient interactions and result in differential care.[96–99] A systematic review found that health-care providers hold implicit racial and ethnic biases, and that these biases were associated with disparities in treatment recommendations and patient–provider communication, expectations, and empathy.[97] Research also suggests that children with public insurance are less likely to be offered an appointment than privately insured children, which may reflect socioeconomic bias.[100] More research on how racism and discrimination in school and health-care systems can contribute to disparities in child sleep and related functional outcomes is needed. In addition, given that delaying school start times can benefit adolescent sleep,[101] more research is needed on how school schedules could contribute to or buffer against sleep health disparities.

Neighborhood Level

Both physical (eg, air quality, green space) and social (eg, safety) characteristics of neighborhoods impact child sleep, including sleep patterns, insomnia symptoms, and SDB.[17] For example, environmental allergens and toxins may lead to increased SDB symptoms via upper airway inflammation.[55,56] As previously mentioned, environmental factors such as light, noise, and community violence may contribute to child and family sleep disruptions.[26,38,79] Although research examining neighborhood factors is growing, mechanistic studies of modifiable determinants are needed.

SUMMARY AND FUTURE DIRECTIONS

The research in this review suggests that there are well-established racial, ethnic, and socioeconomic sleep health disparities from early childhood through adolescence. At the same time, there are notable research gaps. Most research to date has examined Black–White racial disparities, with less research on other racial and ethnic groups. Only a handful of studies have examined sleep in other NIMHD-designated pediatric health disparity populations, such as gender minorities.[102] Even fewer studies have applied an intersectional framework,[103] which is critical for understanding the causes and influences of sleep health disparities among those with multiple marginalized identities. Research is also needed on dimensions of sleep health beyond duration, timing, and sleep behaviors such as bedtime routines. Future research should also examine contributors to disparities in the prevalence and outcomes of other behavioral and medical sleep disorders.

As described in the recent NIH workshop report on sleep health disparities, there is a need for mechanistic studies, particularly regarding the role of racism and discrimination in these disparities.[3] Interventions that are culturally responsive and address modifiable determinants at multiple socio-ecological levels are also urgently needed.[3] The vast majority of pediatric sleep interventions have been tested with predominantly White families and/or those with higher educational levels.[104] To avoid perpetuating research-to-practice gaps, future research should focus on adapting and evaluating evidence-based interventions in collaboration with health disparity populations and in accessible care settings.[105] Community-engaged research strategies, such as community-based participatory research,[3,105] as well as qualitative and mixed methods, and racial and ethnic health equity principles[106] should be incorporated in both interventional and mechanistic research seeking to address pediatric sleep health disparities.

CLINICS CARE POINTS

- Clinicians should assess for and incorporate multilevel (ie, child, family, school, health-care system, neighborhood, and sociocultural) social and environmental factors when conducting pediatric sleep evaluation, case conceptualization, and treatment-planning.

- Focusing on modifiable social and environmental determinants of sleep health disparities can guide equitable sleep health promotion efforts.

- Clinical training and practice in pediatric sleep should include approaches to reduce implicit and explicit bias and to enhance equitable, culturally humble, and family-centered care.

DECLARATION OF INTERESTS

Dr A.A. Williamson is funded by grants from the National Child Health and Human Development (K23HD094905) and the National Heart, Lung, and Blood Institute (R01HL152454). The authors have no other funding sources or conflicts of interest to disclose.

REFERENCES

1. Minority health, health disparities. Definitions and parameters. NIMHD. Available at: https://www.nimhd.nih.gov/about/strategic-plan/nih-strategic-plan-definitions-and-parameters.html. Accessed March 25, 2022.

2. Boyd RW, Lindo EG, Weeks LD, et al. On racism: a new standard for publishing on racial health inequities. Bethesda, MD: E-publication; 2020. https://doi.org/10.1377/forefront.20200630.939347.

3. Jackson CL, Walker JR, Brown MK, et al. A workshop report on the causes and consequences of sleep health disparities. Sleep 2020; 43(8):zsaa037.

4. Bronfenbrenner U. Ecological systems theory. In: Vasta R, editor. *Six theories of child development: revised formulations and current issues*. London, England: Jessica Kingsley Publishers; 1992. p. 187–249.

5. Buysse DJ. Sleep health: can we define it? Does it matter? Sleep 2014;37(1):9–17.

6. Meltzer LJ, Williamson AA, Mindell JA. Pediatric sleep health: it matters, and so does how we define it. Sleep Med Rev 2021;57:101425.

7. Meltzer LJ, Johnson C, Crosette J, et al. Prevalence of diagnosed sleep disorders in pediatric primary care practices. Pediatrics 2011;125:e1410–8.

8. Ash T, Taveras EM, Redline S, et al. Contextual and parenting factors contribute to shorter sleep among hispanic/latinx compared to non-hispanic white infants. Ann Behav Med 2021;55(5):424–35.

9. Ash T, Davison KK, Haneuse S, et al. Emergence of racial/ethnic differences in infant sleep duration in the first six months of life. Sleep Med X 2019;1: 100003.

10. Lucchini M, Kyle M, Pini N, et al. Racial/ethnic disparities in sleep in mothers and infants during the Covid-19 pandemic. Sleep Health 2022;8(5): 429–39.

11. Nevarez MD, Rifas-Shiman SL, Kleinman KP, et al. Associations of early life risk factors with infant sleep duration. Acad Pediatr 2010;10(3):187–93.

12. Peña MM, Rifas-Shiman SL, Gillman MW, et al. Racial/ethnic and socio-contextual correlates of chronic sleep curtailment in childhood. Sleep 2016;39(9):1653–61.

13. Zhang Z, Adamo KB, Ogden N, et al. Longitudinal correlates of sleep duration in young children. Sleep Med 2021;78:128–34.

14. Smith JP, Hardy ST, Hale LE, et al. Racial disparities and sleep among preschool aged children: a systematic review. Sleep Health 2019;5(1):49–57.

15. Yu X, Quante M, Rueschman M, et al. Emergence of racial/ethnic and socioeconomic differences in objectively measured sleep–wake patterns in early infancy: results of the Rise & SHINE study. Sleep 2021;44(3):zsaa193.

16. Lobermeier M, Staples AD, Peterson C, et al. Cumulative risk, infant sleep, and infant social-emotional development. Infant Behav Dev 2022;67:101713.

17. Mayne SL, Mitchell JA, Virudachalam S, et al. Neighborhood environments and sleep among children and adolescents: a systematic review. Sleep Med Rev 2021;57:101465.

18. Williamson AA, Gould R, Leichman ES, et al. Socioeconomic disadvantage and sleep in early childhood: real-world data from a mobile health application. Sleep Health 2021;7(2):143–52.

19. Grimes M, Camerota M, Propper CB. Neighborhood deprivation predicts infant sleep quality. Sleep Health 2019;5(2):148–51.

20. Hale L, Berger LM, LeBourgeois MK, et al. Social and demographic predictors of preschoolers' bedtime routines. J Dev Behav Pediatr 2009; 30(5):394–402.

21. Williamson AA, Mindell JA. Cumulative sociodemographic risk factors and sleep outcomes in early childhood. Sleep 2020;43(3):zsz233.

22. Guglielmo D, Gazmararian JA, Chung J, et al. Racial/ethnic sleep disparities in US school-aged children and adolescents: a review of the literature. Sleep Health 2018;4(1):68–80.

23. Yip T, Cheon YM, Wang Y, et al. Sociodemographic and environmental factors associated with childhood sleep duration. Sleep Health 2020;6(6):767–77.

24. Jarrin DC, McGrath JJ, Quon EC. Objective and subjective socioeconomic gradients exist for sleep in children and adolescents. Health Psychol 2014; 33(3):301–5.

25. Sheehan C, Powers D, Margerison-Zilko C, et al. Historical neighborhood poverty trajectories and child sleep. Sleep Health 2018;4(2):127–34.

26. El-Sheikh M, Bagley EJ, Keiley M, et al. Economic adversity and children's sleep problems: multiple indicators and moderation of effects. Health Psychol 2013;32(8):849–59.

27. Marczyk Organek KD, Taylor DJ, Petrie T, et al. Adolescent sleep disparities: sex and racial/ethnic differences. Sleep Health 2015;1(1):36–9.

28. Yip T, Cheon YM, Wang Y, et al. Racial disparities in sleep: associations with discrimination among ethnic/racial minority adolescents. Child Dev 2020;91(3):914–31.

29. James S, Chang AM, Buxton OM, et al. Disparities in adolescent sleep health by sex and ethnoracial group. SSM Popul Health 2020;11:100581.

30. Matthews KA, Hall M, Dahl RE. Sleep in healthy black and white adolescents. Pediatrics 2014; 133(5):e1189–96.

31. Marco CA, Wolfson AR, Sparling M, et al. Family socioeconomic status and sleep patterns of young adolescents. Behav Sleep Med 2012;10(1):70–80.

32. El-Sheikh M, Shimizu M, Philbrook LE, et al. Sleep and development in adolescence in the context of socioeconomic disadvantage. J Adolesc 2020; 83(1):1–11.

33. Milan S, Snow S, Belay S. The context of preschool children's sleep: racial/ethnic differences in sleep locations, routines, and concerns. J Fam Psychol 2007;21(1):20–8.

34. Patrick KE, Millet G, Mindell JA. Sleep differences by race in preschool children: the roles of parenting behaviors and socioeconomic status. Behav Sleep Med 2015;14(5):467–79.

35. Owens JA, Spirito A, McGuinn M, et al. Sleep habits and sleep disturbance in elementary school-aged children. J Dev Behav Pediatr 2000;21(1):27–36.

36. Sheares BJ, Kattan M, Leu CS, et al. Sleep problems in urban, minority, early-school-aged children more prevalent than previously recognized. Clin Pediatr 2013;52(4):302–9.

37. Rubens SL, Patrick KE, Williamson AA, et al. Individual and socio-demographic factors related to presenting problem and diagnostic impressions at a pediatric sleep clinic. Sleep Med 2016;25: 67–72.

38. Bagley EJ, Kelly RJ, Buckhalt JA, et al. What keeps low-SES children from sleeping well: the role of pre-sleep worries and sleep environment. Sleep Med 2015;16(4):496–502.

39. El-Sheikh M, Philbrook LE, Kelly RJ, et al. What does a good night's sleep mean? Nonlinear relations between sleep and children's cognitive functioning and mental health. Sleep 2019;42(6): zsz078.

40. Fernandez-Mendoza J, Bourchtein E, Calhoun S, et al. Natural history of insomnia symptoms in the transition from childhood to adolescence: population rates, health disparities, and risk factors. Sleep 2021;44(3):zsaa187.

41. Troxel WM, Shih RA, Ewing B, et al. Examination of neighborhood disadvantage and sleep in a multi-ethnic cohort of adolescents. Health Place 2017; 45:39–45.

42. Zapata Roblyer MI, Grzywacz J. Demographic and parenting correlates of adolescent sleep functioning. J Child Fam Stud 2015;24(11):3331–40.

43. Roberts RE, Roberts CR, Chan W. Ethnic differences in symptoms of insomnia among adolescents. Sleep 2006;29(3):359–65.

44. Roberts RE, Lee ES, Hemandez M, et al. Symptoms of insomnia among adolescents in the lower Rio Grande Valley of Texas. Sleep 2004;27(4): 751–60.

45. Bixler EO, Vgontzas AN, Lin HM, et al. Sleep disordered breathing in children in a general population sample: prevalence and risk factors. Sleep 2009; 32(6):6.

46. Rosen CL, Larkin EK, Kirchner HL, et al. Prevalence and risk factors for sleep-disordered breathing in 8- to 11-year-old children: association with race and prematurity. J Pediatr 2003;142(4):383–9.

47. Montgomery-Downs HE, Gozal D. Sleep habits and risk factors for sleep-disordered breathing in infants and young toddlers in Louisville, Kentucky. Sleep Med 2006;7(3):211–9.

48. Goldstein NA, Abramowitz T, Weedon J, et al. Racial/ethnic differences in the prevalence of snoring and sleep disordered breathing in young children. J Clin Sleep Med 2011;7(2):163–71.

49. Brouillette RT, Horwood L, Constantin E, et al. Childhood sleep apnea and neighborhood disadvantage. J Pediatr 2011;158(5):789–95.e1.

50. Archbold KH, Pituch KJ, Panahi P, et al. Symptoms of sleep disturbances among children at two general pediatric clinics. J Pediatr 2002;140(1): 97–102.

51. Marcus CL, Brooks LJ, Draper KA, et al. Diagnosis and management of childhood obstructive sleep apnea syndrome. Pediatrics 2012;130(3):576–84.

52. Redline S, Tishler PV, Schluchter M, et al. Risk factors for sleep-disordered breathing in children: associations with obesity, race, and respiratory problems. Am J Respir Crit Care Med 1999; 159(5):1527–32.

53. Weinstock TG, Rosen CL, Marcus CL, et al. Predictors of obstructive sleep apnea severity in adeno-tonsillectomy candidates. Sleep 2014;37(2):261–9.

54. Boss EF, Smith DF, Ishman SL. Racial/ethnic and socioeconomic disparities in the diagnosis and treatment of sleep-disordered breathing in children. Int J Pediatr Otorhinolaryngol 2011;75(3): 299–307.

55. Spilsbury JC, Storfer-Isser A, Kirchner HL, et al. Neighborhood disadvantage as a risk factor for pediatric obstructive sleep apnea. J Pediatr 2006; 149(3):342–7.

56. Wang R, Dong Y, Weng J, et al. Associations among neighborhood, race, and sleep apnea severity in children. A six-city analysis. Ann Am Thorac Soc 2017;14(1):76–84.

57. Cooper JN, Koppera S, Boss EF, et al. Differences in tonsillectomy utilization by race/ethnicity, type of health insurance, and rurality. Acad Pediatr 2021; 21(6):1031–6.

58. Kum-Nji P, Mangrem CL, Wells PJ, et al. Black/white differential use of health services by young

children in a rural Mississippi community. South Med J 2006;99(9):957–62.

59. Marcus CL, Moore RH, Rosen CL, et al. A randomized trial of adenotonsillectomy for childhood sleep apnea. N Engl J Med 2013;368(25):2366–76.

60. Pecha PP, Chew M, Andrews AL. Racial and ethnic disparities in utilization of tonsillectomy among medicaid-insured children. J Pediatr 2021;233: 191–7.e2.

61. Boss EF, Benke JR, Tunkel DE, et al. Public insurance and timing of polysomnography and surgical care for children with sleep-disordered breathing. JAMA Otolaryngol-Head Neck Surg 2015;141(2): 106–11.

62. Billings ME, Cohen RT, Baldwin CM, et al. Disparities in sleep health and potential intervention models. Chest 2021;159(3):1232–40.

63. Williamson AA, Johnson TJ, Tapia IE. Health disparities in pediatric sleep-disordered breathing. Paediatr Respir Rev 2022;S1526-0542(22):00005–7.

64. Paradies Y, Ben J, Denson N, et al. Racism as a determinant of health: a systematic review and meta-analysis. PLoS One 2015;10(9):e0138511.

65. Pieterse AL, Todd NR, Neville HA, et al. Perceived racism and mental health among Black American adults: a meta-analytic review. J Couns Psychol 2012;59(1):1–9.

66. Trent M, Dooley DG, Dougé J, et al. The impact of racism on child and adolescent health. Pediatrics 2019;144(2):e20191765.

67. Berry OO, Londoño Tobón A, Njoroge WFM. Social determinants of health: the impact of racism on early childhood mental health. Curr Psychiatry Rep 2021;23(5):23.

68. Sadeh A, Tikotzky L, Scher A. Parenting and infant sleep. Sleep Med Rev 2010;14(2):89–96.

69. Sadeh A, Anders TF. Infant sleep problems: origins, assessment, interventions. Infant Ment Health J 1993;14(1):17–34.

70. Jian N, Teti DM. Emotional availability at bedtime, infant temperament, and infant sleep development from one to six months. Sleep Med 2016;23:49–58.

71. Fuller-Rowell TE, Nichols OI, Burrow AL, et al. Day-to-day fluctuations in experiences of discrimination: associations with sleep and the moderating role of internalized racism among African American college students. Cultur Divers Ethnic Minor Psychol 2021;27(1):107–17.

72. Goosby BJ, Cheadle JE, Strong-Bak W, et al. Perceived discrimination and adolescent sleep in a community sample. RSF 2018;4(4):43–61.

73. Huynh VW, Gillen-O'Neel C. Discrimination and sleep: the protective role of school belonging. Youth Soc 2016;48(5):649–72.

74. Bathory E, Tomopoulos S, Rothman R, et al. Infant sleep and parent health literacy. Acad Pediatr 2016;16(6):550–7.

75. Owens JA, Jones C. Parental knowledge of healthy sleep in young children: results of a primary care clinic survey. J Dev Behav Pediatr 2011;32(6): 447–53.

76. Cespedes EM, Gillman MW, Kleinman K, et al. Television viewing, bedroom television, and sleep duration from infancy to mid-childhood. Pediatrics 2014;133(5):e1163–71.

77. Palimaru AI, Dong L, Brown RA, et al. Mental health, family functioning, and sleep in cultural context among American Indian/Alaska native urban youth: a mixed methods analysis. Soc Sci Med 2022;292:114582.

78. Quante M, Khandpur N, Kontos EZ, et al. Let's talk about sleep": a qualitative examination of levers for promoting healthy sleep among sleep-deprived vulnerable adolescents. Sleep Med 2019;60:81–8.

79. Wilson KE, Miller AL, Bonuck K, et al. Sleep environments and sleep durations in a sample of low-income preschool children. J Clin Sleep Med 2014;10(3):7.

80. Mileva-Seitz VR, Bakersmans-Kraneburg MJ, Battaini C, et al. Parent-child bed-sharing: the good, the bad, and the burden of evidence. Sleep Med Rev 2017;32:4–27.

81. Covington LB, Armstrong B, Black MM. Bed sharing in toddlerhood: choice versus necessity and provider guidelines. Glob Pediatr Health 2019;6. https://doi.org/10.1177/2333794X19843929. 2333794X19843929.

82. Mindell JA, Sadeh A, Wiegand B, et al. Cross-cultural differences in infant and toddler sleep. Sleep Med 2010;11(3):274–80.

83. Barajas RG, Martin A, Brooks-Gunn J, et al. Mother-child bed-sharing in toddlerhood and cognitive and behavioral outcomes. Pediatrics 2011;128(2): e339–47.

84. Zambrano DN, Mindell JA, Reyes NR, et al. It's not all about my baby's sleep": a qualitative study of factors influencing low-income african american mothers' sleep quality. Behav Sleep Med 2016; 14(5):489–500.

85. Caldwell BA, Ordway MR, Sadler LS, et al. Parent perspectives on sleep and sleep habits among young children living with economic adversity. J Pediatr Health Care 2020;34(1):10–22.

86. Williamson AA, Milaniak I, Watson B, et al. Early childhood sleep intervention in urban primary care: caregiver and clinician perspectives. J Pediatr Psychol 2020;45(8):933–45.

87. Spilsbury JC, Patel SR, Morris N, et al. Household chaos and sleep-disturbing behavior of family members: results of a pilot study of African American early adolescents. Sleep Health 2017;3(2): 84–9.

88. Koopman-Verhoeff ME, Serdarevic F, Kocevska D, et al. Preschool family irregularity and the

development of sleep problems in childhood: a longitudinal study. J Child Psychol Psychiatry 2019; 60(8):856–7.

89. Covington LB, Patterson F, Hale LE, et al. The contributory role of the family context in early childhood sleep health: a systematic review. Sleep Health 2021;7(2):254–65.

90. Daniel LC, Childress JL, Flannery JL, et al. Identifying modifiable factors linking parenting and sleep in racial/ethnic minority children. J Pediatr Psychol 2020;45(8):867–76.

91. Fronberg KM, Bai S, Teti DM. Household chaos mediates the link between family resources and child sleep. Sleep Health 2022;8:121–9.

92. Rojo-Wissar DM, Owusu JT, Nyhuis C, et al. Parent-child relationship quality and sleep among adolescents: modification by race/ethnicity. Sleep Health 2020;6(2):145–52.

93. Powell CA, Rifas-Shiman SL, Oken E, et al. Maternal experiences of racial discrimination and offspring sleep in the first 2 years of life: project Viva cohort, Massachusetts, USA (1999-2002). Sleep Health 2020;6(4):463–8.

94. Slopen N, Lewis TT, Williams DR. Discrimination and sleep: a systematic review. Sleep Med Rev 2016;18:88–95.

95. Cohen MF, Dunlop AL, Johnson DA, et al. Intergenerational effects of discrimination on black american children's sleep health. Int J Environ Res Public Health 2022;19(7):4021.

96. Blackson EA, Gerdes M, Segan E, et al. Racial bias toward children in the early childhood education setting. J Early Child Res 2022. https://doi.org/10.1177/1476718X221087051. 1476718X221087051.

97. Maina IW, Belton TD, Ginzberg S, et al. A decade of studying implicit racial/ethnic bias in healthcare providers using the implicit association test. Soc Sci Med 2018;199:219–29.

98. Starck JG, Riddle T, Sinclair S, et al. Teachers are people too: examining the racial bias of teachers compared to other american adults. Educ Res 2020;49(4):273–84.

99. van Ryn M. Research on the provider contribution to race/ethnicity disparities in medical care. Med Care 2002;40:I140–51.

100. Wang EC, Choe MC, Meara JG, et al. Inequality of access to surgical specialty health care: why children with government-funded insurance have less access than those with private insurance in Southern California. Pediatrics 2004;114(5):e584–90.

101. Yip T, Wang Y, Xie M, et al. School Start Times, Sleep, and Youth Outcomes: A Meta-analysis. Pediatrics 2022;149(6):e2021054068.

102. Levenson JC, Thoma BC, Hamilton JL, et al. Sleep among gender minority adolescents. Sleep 2021; 44(3):zsaa185.

103. Crenshaw K. Demarginalizing the intersection of race and sex: A black feminist critique of antidiscrimination doctrine, feminist theory and antiracist politics. University of Chicago Legal Forum 1989, no. 1 (1989): 139-167.

104. Schwichtenberg AJ, Abel EA, Keys E, et al. Diversity in pediatric behavioral sleep intervention studies. Sleep Med Rev 2019;47:103–11.

105. Baumann AA, Cabassa LJ. Reframing implementation science to address inequities in healthcare delivery. BMC Health Serv Res 2020;20(1):190.

106. Andrews K, Parekh J, Peckoo S. How to embed a racial and ethnic equity perspective in research: practical guidance for the research process. Child Trends 2019. Available at: https://www.researchconnections.org/childcare/resources/38276. Accessed May 2, 2022.

Sleep Technology

David G. Ingram, MD, MHPE*, Tamika A. Cranford, MHPE, RRT-NPS, RPSGT, CCSH,
Baha Al-Shawwa, MD

KEYWORDS

- Technology • Pediatric sleep • Polysomnography • Home sleep testing • Pulse-wave analysis
- Wearables

KEY POINTS

- Electroencephalogram (EEG) spectral analysis and measures of autonomic activity such as pulse-wave amplitude may provide complementary information compared with traditional sleep staging.
- Home sleep testing for pediatric obstructive sleep apnea is not yet standard of care but remains an active area of research.
- A multitude of consumer sleep technologies are available including wearables for the management of sleep and breathing, interventional devices, and smartphone applications.
- Readers are directed to SleepTechnology on the American Academy of Sleep Medicine (AASM) website as an excellent up-to-date resource on consumer sleep technology.

INTRODUCTION

A thorough understanding of technology related to sleep in children is necessary for practicing pediatric sleep providers. Signal acquisition, sensor issues, and other aspects of standard polysomnography frequently require troubleshooting and mastery for physicians to render accurate sleep study interpretation. In addition, it is widely recognized that our traditional metrics derived from standard polysomnography, although providing a starting point in a young field, may not fully capture the possible data that can be derived from polysomnography and that novel measures under development may better characterize sleep phenotype and disorders. Finally, sleep providers are often tasked with interpreting information derived from consumer sleep devices as well as advising families on the potential utility of such technologies in their child's care. In this review, we discuss the opportunities and challenges of technology as it relates to the pediatric sleep clinic.

DISCUSSION

Successfully Performing Polysomnography in Children

Performing sleep studies in children requires a unique skill set and approach compared with adults. In our experience, a child's age alone is not a reliable predictor of how smoothly a sleep study will proceed. Although a healthy 2-year-old may sit perfectly still while being set up, a teenager with neurodevelopmental or sensory disorders may have significant meltdowns. As a countermeasure, we commonly employ distraction in the form of toys, tablets, and television. Sometimes a difficult set up requires multiple technologists. For example, while the parent holds the child in their lap, one technologist can blow bubbles playing with them whereas the other is attaching sensors. In addition, when available, a child life team can be invaluable in assisting with different types of distractions during this time. The help of child life has frequently been a deciding factor in the success of a set up, and without them, the study would either have not been completed or it would have taken much longer and been a much bigger ordeal. Indeed, our anecdotal experiences are reinforced by published work utilizing the Six Sigma framework, which identified multiple interventions to enhance patient and family experience in the pediatric sleep lab (listed in **Box 1**).[1]

Pediatric sleep studies require carbon dioxide (CO_2) monitoring throughout the study, whether they are placed on positive airway pressure

Division of Pulmonary and Sleep Medicine, Children's Mercy Hospital, 2401 Gillham Road, Kansas City, MO 64108, USA
* Corresponding author.
E-mail address: dgingram@cmh.edu

Sleep Med Clin 18 (2023) 235–244
https://doi.org/10.1016/j.jsmc.2023.01.009
1556-407X/23/

Box 1
Possible interventions for enhancing patient and family experience in the pediatric sleep lab according to a study by Baughn and colleagues[1]

- Patient appointment guide
- FAQs document
- Informational video from child's perspective
- Empathic communication training
- Check billing requirements to see if the child must be present for a follow-up consult
- Allow early check-ins
- Be flexible with the number of parents present for bedtime needs
- Make waiting areas and sleep rooms child-friendly
- Reduce co-mingled waiting room
- Provide access to a refrigerator
- Offer tours
- Comfortable bed for a parent
- Check-in bags with fun items
- Make family feel like guests
- Consider EEG cap versus leads
- Utilize distraction techniques
- Apply child life practices to help with anxiety
- Set check-out expectations and offer breakfast

(PAP) or not. Children typically do not like the sensation of the cannula in their nose, so we typically place this immediately before we put them to bed. Most kids will leave the cannula in place, but on occasion, it is necessary to wait until they are in delta sleep for placement. In the scenario where cannula placement is unsuccessful or PAP is initiated, we will still place a thermistor wire but will employ a transcutaneous monitor instead for CO_2 measurement. Once set up is complete and impedances are verified less than 5, we will sometimes wrap the patient's head with gauze or Coban to help keep the leads in place. With the Coban, we use the multicolor pack so that the child can pick a color. Finally, we place a sleeve on all the wires to keep the patient from getting tangled in all of them. These two approaches help reduce the need for the technologist to re-enter the room to readjust sensors.

Bedtime can sometimes be a challenge for families in the sleep lab. A portion of patients still sleep in a crib, which we have available, whereas others sleep in a toddler bed (we use rails along both

sides of the bed) or a standard bed. Occasionally children prefer to sleep on their own, whereas others need a parental presence for sleep onset. In the latter scenario, we allow the parent to lay in the bed with the child until they fall asleep and then have them move to the parent's bed. This can make for a difficult night for the parent if they are moving in and out of the bed when the child wakes during the night. When the parent is in the room, they are educated that they must be as quiet as possible and have electronics turned off, as any noise can affect the study. If the parent is not ready to sleep, we direct them to a separate parent room and request they check with the technologist before re-entering in case the patient is in Rapid eye movement sleep (REM).

Even if the initial set up goes smoothly, there can be multiple issues to troubleshoot throughout the night. As a rule, always check the patient first. The oximeter may consistently read 100% or have inadequate waveform. It is important to check for common issues that affect oximetry accuracy including that the oximeter probe is not being pulled and still flush with the toe or finger, that the patient's appendage is not cold (as the rooms are kept cool to help prevent sweating), and that it is not being laid on. An effort belt may go in and out due to the belt being twisted. The child may have been playing with it and severed the connection. Make sure the belt did not come undone, is still plugged into the headbox, and check the buckle. If those are intact, replace the belt strip, and if it is still not functioning, replace the buckle apparatus.

When having problems with head leads, look to see if there is a pattern in the disruption. Press on the M leads to make sure they are well attached and add more paste if needed. With one lead popping, check and add the paste. Sometimes, the site needs to be cleaned again, the new paste applied, and tape or gauze square. If this approach does not result in a fix, replace the wire. In the case where the patient is sweating excessively during sleep, this can result in sway in the EEG. To help in this scenario, try flipping the patient's pillow over, use some alcohol on a 4x4, and dab it on the patient's head where the leads are placed or use a small fan pointed at the patient's head.

Lastly, if the pressure transducer/end-tidal carbon dioxide (ETCO2)/thermistor quit working, first ensure that it is still in the patient's nose. If the pressure transducer is working but not the ETCO2 (or vice versa), try switching the ends (headbox and ETCO2 machine) to see if this resolves the issue. It could be that the child is mouth breathing, in which case switching to an oronasal cannula will help. If it was a difficult set up and the child cried most of the time, there could be secretions blocking the cannula, and it is necessary to replace the cannula to obtain an adequate signal. Consider cutting the cannula and placing a new one and taping it down without waking the child. The best time to be in the room to fix or replace items is generally during delta sleep.

Novel Metrics Derived from Standard Polysomnography

Electroencephalogram (EEG) analysis

EEG signals obtained from limited scalp points (central, occipital, and frontal) have been the gold standard in identifying EEG activity during a polysomnogram. The current method of scoring sleep stages and awakenings utilizes visual characteristics on a 30-second epoch but does not quantify EEG activity. The advances in technology and computing power have provided the means to quantify EEG activity, revealing information about the quality of sleep beyond sleep staging. Many of the current sleep software systems have the ability of "spectral analysis," quantifying EEG power activity such as delta (1–4 Hz), theta (4–8 Hz), alpha (8–12 Hz), sigma (12–15 Hz), and beta (15–30 Hz), although this is not currently widely used for clinical purposes. The delineation of spectral activity holds promise for exposing additional meaningful information. For example, delta activity reflects the homeostatic process of sleep and is usually highest at the beginning of the night when the need for recuperation is greatest. Previous research has shown that delta sleep is increased following extended awakenings[2] and decreased in sleep following a daytime nap.[3]

EEG spectral power analyses have been used to identify a variety of EEG characteristics in disease processes. For example, higher frequency EEG signal (such as beta) within sleep reflects an arousal state and is often increased in insomnia.[4] In contrast, lower delta power has been found in patients with psychiatric disorders such as schizophrenia.[5] In pediatric patients with obstructive sleep apnea (OSA), a study has shown that OSA episodes without cortical arousals significantly decrease the delta power and is followed by rebound upon the termination of the respiratory event.[6] Subsequent analysis from that spectral analysis of EEG provides complementary information and may be able to better elucidate OSA phenotype in children.[7]

Noninvasive autonomic signals

In addition to sleep staging, a polysomnogram EEG signal remains the gold standard in detecting arousals and awakenings. However, there is increasing research showing arousals being identified non-invasively through other readily available autonomic markers. These markers are presented as changes in cardiovascular measures including heart rate, blood pressure, peripheral arterial tonometry (PAT), pulse transit time (PTT), pulse-wave velocity, and pulse-wave amplitude (PWA).[8–13] Earlier studies demonstrated that arousals associated with OSA produce cyclic changes in heart rate, and another study showed tactile arousal stimulus increased noninvasive beat-to-beat blood pressure.[9,10] Furthermore, children are less likely to show EEG cortical arousals compared with adults in response to different stimuli, including sleep-disordered breathing.[14] Therefore, it is prudent to find more sensitive ways of identifying arousals in children. PTT is a calculated measure obtained from the electrocardiogram and finger pulse signals of the pulse oximetry. It has been shown that PTT is a very sensitive measure for subcortical/autonomic arousals, even in children.[8,15]

Another related measure of interest is PWA, which is a signal obtained from finger photoplethysmography and is strongly correlated to finger blood flow. A drop in the PWA signal is a marker for finger vasoconstriction that is shown to be a very sensitive marker for subcortical/autonomic arousals (**Fig. 1**). In addition, a recent study showed that the drop in PWA could help in guiding scoring respiratory events and children.[16] The study showed that using a PWA drop signal as a surrogate marker for arousals substantially affected the hypopnea scoring and increased the severity of OSA from mild (obstructive apnea-hypopnea index [AHI] index between 1 and 5 events per hour) to moderate (obstructive AHI index between 5 and 10 events per hour) in about 50% of the patients studied. Similarly, PAT is another measure that is widely studied and serves as the basis for some home sleep apnea tests. Algorithms utilize changes in PAT in conjunction with oxygen desaturation, heart rate changes, snoring, and body position to identify respiratory events, sleep/wake status, and estimate sleep stages.

Investigative Technology for Sleep Measurement

Home sleep apnea testing

Clinicians caring for children who have clinical sleep problems are often evaluating for the possibility of OSA as a contributor to their sleep challenges. As such, polysomnography is a routinely utilized tool as a part of the evaluation and management of these patients. Unfortunately, the supply of qualified pediatric sleep providers as well as the limited number and beds and pediatric sleep

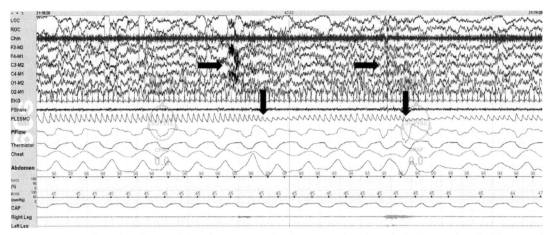

Fig. 1. A 60-second window from in-lab polysomnography demonstrating drops in PWA associated with arousals. Drops in the PWA signal may be a sensitive marker of subcortical/autonomic arousals to help identify respiratory events in conjunction with diminution in airflow.

laboratories limits the availability of this resource and results and potentially prolonged wait times for patients and families. In-lab polysomnography is also resource intensive with the need for technologists which are experienced and adept at working with children who often have neurodevelopmental disorders and other complex medical conditions. In addition, the setting of a sleep lab is a different environment than the home setting, which can result in potentially different findings on sleep testing. For these reasons, there has been intense interest in developing and validating a home sleep apnea test (HSAT) that can accurately provide supportive or refute evidence for the diagnosis of sleep-related breathing disorders in children.

One important issue relating to assessing the diagnostic adequacy of home sleep testing is a firm understanding of performance metrics. This issue was illustrated very nicely in a recent paper by Massie and colleagues.[17] The authors point out the important distinction between correlation coefficients and diagnostic concordance. Although correlation coefficients can assess if two measurements are linearly related, this can sometimes be quite misleading and not accurately reflect diagnostic accuracy. In contrast, the more clinically prescient performance metric of diagnostic accuracy or concordance reflects the percentage agreement of diagnostic category. When the authors performed a meta-analysis of the literature to compare these metrics, they found that overall, there was a high correlation between HSAT and in-lab polysomnography apnea-hypopnea indices of 0.82, but the average diagnostic accuracy was only 0.61 with an overall misdiagnosis rate of 39%. Furthermore, the

authors observed a large underreporting of diagnostic accuracy metrics in published papers, with only 6 out of 20 papers directly reporting diagnostic accuracy. Overall, the study highlights the need for clinicians to carefully review reported accuracy performance measures from studies so they can be applied appropriately in the clinical setting, as failure to do so may result in unintended diagnostic conclusions and management decisions.

The American Academy of Sleep Medicine brought together experts in pediatric sleep medicine in 2017 to publish a position paper on the use of HSAT in children.[18] The task force performed a review of the literature available at the time and overall concluded that HSAT was not recommended for the diagnosis OSA in children but left the final judgment to the discretion of the treating clinician considering available diagnostic tools and treatment options within their clinical context. The task force also identified challenges unique to home testing in children, including adequate identification of arousals and hypoventilation, application of home studies in children with significant comorbidities as well as very young children, variation and body size across the age range, and individual caregiver ability to properly navigate sensors during the night in the home setting.

Since the publication of that position paper, work has continued in this space to address the limitations of previous studies. Masoud and colleagues[19] examined the potential diagnostic value of a portable sleep monitor (which included chest and abdominal effort bands, nasal cannula pressure transducer, finger pulse oximetry sensor, microphone, and body position sensor) in children at their center and found a high sensitivity and specificity for the ability of the device to detect severe sleep apnea, operationalized as an AHI greater than or equal to 10/hour. A very large and recent study that was performed examined over 500 healthy 1-year-old Canadian infants utilizing home sleep cardiorespiratory monitoring. That study reported on reference data for healthy infants that could potentially be used for normative comparison, although it did not have in-lab polysomnography for comparison.[20] Home sleep testing was examined in a sample of adolescents with neuromuscular disorders, and although HSAT was preferred by patients, it was unable to definitively rule out sleep-disordered breathing and underestimated the AHI by an average of 10/hour.[21] The potential utility of adding in PTT along with respiratory polygraphy was examined in a group of children aged 3 to 17 years with a wide range of disease severity, and the authors found preliminarily supportive results with improved diagnostic accuracy (good agreement on Bland Altman plot), including adequate identification of hypopneas.[22] Highlighting the potential challenges with sensor application in the home setting, a recent study found that only 53% of recordings were successfully obtained in HSAT in children, mainly related to signal failure with a nasal cannula, pulse oximetry, and battery failure; failure rates were improved by using simple sensor fixation techniques.[23] A recent prospective study evaluating an HSAT device and questionnaire in children found that although 85% were able to obtain adequate data for the home test, there was a very large difference in results with a mean difference of 14/hour with wide confidence intervals for AHI compared to in-lab polysomnography.[24] Recent studies suggest that providing an online video attending technician or telehealth support during the HSAT in children can be beneficial for testing success in the home environment.[25,26]

Home sleep apnea testing distinct from respiratory polygraphy methods has also been investigated. Overnight pulse oximetry has long been studied as a potential screening tool for OSA and children. A recent diagnostic meta-analysis found that pulse oximetry had pooled sensitivities and specificities of 0.5 and 0.8 for an AHI great than 1/hour, 0.8 and 0.7 for an AHI greater than 5/hour, and 0.8 and 0.8 for an AHI greater than 10/hour.[27] An important limitation of overnight oximetry in the home setting that clinicians should be aware of is a substantial night-to-night variability that is clinically meaningful in magnitude.[28] Pulse oximetry signal quality is significantly lower as compared to that obtained in the hospital setting, possibly related to movement artifact.[29] PAT technology has some theoretic advantages including the absence of nasal pressure transducer and respiratory effort belts that could potentially increase tolerability, although its ability to mimic diagnostic accuracy of in-lab studies to date has been variable.[30–32] A particularly promising and novel system has recently been studied and includes a noninvasive mattress system that has encased within it multiple sensors that detect body movement as well as breathing sounds to derive continuous metrics of obstructive sleep-disordered breathing during sleep. This device is able to accurately detect and classify obstructive and central respiratory events and estimate the apnea–hypopnea index.[33] More importantly, the device allows for quantification of partial airway obstruction, characterized by snoring and stertor that are not captured by the current scoring criteria. These episodes of airway obstruction may be associated with a greater degree of sleep disruption than apneas and hypopneas,[34] identify episodes of obstructive hypoventilation,[35] and be a more sensitive marker of treatment efficacy than AHI alone.[36]

Consumer technology considerations

The consumer sleep device field is a rapidly evolving space of clinical import. Given the widespread availability and use of devices that can be purchased by families over the counter, as well as applications that can be downloaded for smartphone use, sleep medicine providers are frequently tasked with evaluating questions and data from patients and families who have utilized these technologies. Given the substantial challenges that this poses for sleep health care providers, the AASM Consumer and Clinical Technology committee published a position statement in 2018 that discussed the potential advantages and disadvantages of consumer sleep technology for clinicians.[37] Since that time, they went on to develop and maintain a novel online resource for members called #SleepTechnology on the AASM website, available here: https://aasm.org/consumer-clinical-sleep-technology/. This incredibly helpful resource provides an up-to-date summary of device capabilities, derived metrics, type of platform, FDA status, mechanism of measurement, and any available peer-reviewed publications. The website currently lists reviews of well over 100 different consumer sleep technologies, and the reader is directed to this resource for the most up-to-date information regarding any particular device or technology.

Sleep and breathing measurement

Many wrist-worn band devices have been developed to estimate sleep.[38–42] A major limitation of wrist-worn devices based on movement alone is their inability to accurately and reliably detect wake after sleep onset. A meta-analysis found that the accuracy of even research-grade actigraphy devices is substantially influenced by device and child-specific characteristics.[43] One recent study performed in children examining a commercially available device, clinical actigraphy, and polysomnography found that the commercially available device provided similar or even better agreement with polysomnography compared with actigraphy.[44] Wristwatch-based sensors have also been developed that can measure oxygen saturation and heart rate, as well as estimate sleep based on heart rate variability and motion.[45] Multiple devices designed to be worn on the finger as a band with built-in pulse oximetry have been developed to capture patterns to estimate sleep parameters including sleep architecture and AHI.[46–48] One fascinating device analyzes the pulse oximetry signal from a cardiopulmonary coupling basis. The software estimates an apnea-hypopnea index, but also intriguingly reports other sleep architecture metrics including a novel sleep quality index and a 3D spectrogram based on cardiopulmonary coupling principles. This approach has been specifically evaluated in both adults as well as children with some promising results.[49–52] Pulse oximeters specifically designed for infants have also been introduced into the consumer market intended for home use monitoring.[53,54] Analysis of mandibular movement during sleep has been examined as a method to diagnose sleep apnea, and one study in children specifically showed a promising ability to diagnose moderate to severe pediatric OSA.[55] Some devices have been constructed that can be placed underneath a sleeping surface to measure parameters such as heart rate, breathing, and estimate sleep; the accuracy of such devices is variable.[56] Other devices use radar or sonar technology to monitor breathing and sleep in a noncontact form.[57–59] Some devices with EEG sensors built into the headband have demonstrated impressive results in adults in terms of estimating sleep architecture.[60–62]

Interventional devices

Alternative treatments for OSA have also been investigated. One device is designed to be worn around the front of the neck and provides negative air pressure to help alleviate upper airway obstruction.[63] Another device has been developed that provides neuromuscular electrical stimulation to the tongue while awake, with the idea that this can induce muscle changes with regular use to help treat sleep-disordered breathing.[64] A novel appliance has been developed that provides intraoral negative air pressure throughout the night to help maintain airway patency.[65] A cooling headband has been invented that is meant to reduce metabolic activity in the frontal cortex and therefore promote sleep by minimizing hyperarousal states; one randomized control trial in adults with insomnia was shown positive results and objectively measured improvement in sleep.[66] Wearable glasses with a built-in lightbox have been created as a form of bright light therapy and found to be beneficial in terms of improving sleepiness and attention[67]; of note, this device was also tested specifically in adolescents with delayed sleep phase syndrome in a randomized controlled trial and found to be of benefit compared with sham device.[68] Drowsy driving is often a safety consideration in patients with sleep disorders, and systems have been developed in which the driver wears glasses to monitor eyelid blinking parameters to identify drowsy driving and alert the driver to avoid falling asleep at the wheel.[69] Some alarm clocks now incorporate a light component to stimulate sunset and dawn with the idea that this can potentially improve mood and energy in the morning upon awakening, with studies showing mixed results.[70–72]

Several devices utilize vibroacoustic stimulation in an attempt to enhance sleep. One device is meant to be placed inside the pillow and then delivers vibrational sound during the course of the night; of note, this device was tested in a pilot study in children with autism spectrum disorder and found to be associated with improved sleep as well as daytime behaviors related to their autism, attention, and quality of life.[73] Another interesting device is a band that is either worn on the wrist or the ankle that provides external vibration at specific frequencies with the idea that it will increase heart rate variability, possibly resulting in a variety of health effects.[74] External vibrations have also been utilized to promote positional therapy for sleep apnea by having patients wear a device that vibrates until the person moves off their back.[75,76] Acoustic auditory stimulation has also been explored as a way to enhance slow-wave sleep and promote more restorative sleep.[77] One non-pharmacologic option that has been explored for restless leg syndrome is a vibratory counter stimulation pad to be used at night, with some promising results in adults.[78] Finally, in terms of insomnia therapy, the concept of intensive sleep retraining is based on the idea that the person is aroused by delivering vibrations during the first hour of sleep to train the body to fall asleep by inducing the sensation of falling asleep over and over again.[79]

Smartphone applications

Manufacturers of PAP devices have developed their smartphone applications to help consumers track PAP-related data including usage, leak, and residual respiratory events. They also can include some educational content for patients.[80,81] Some smartphones and devices can adjust screen colors at night with the idea that this will help with sleep onset and quality, although one study did not show any significant effects on melatonin secretion.[82] Applications have been created that can analyze sounds throughout the night and attempt to identify abnormal breathing patterns.[83] Other smartphone applications attempt to quantify sleep and sleep architecture from measurements of movement, sonar, and noise.[84–86] Given the paucity of behavioral sleep psychologists, it is no surprise that an application has been developed to help deliver cognitive behavioral therapy for insomnia, with positive results from randomized control trials in adults.[87,88]

SUMMARY

Sleep technology is a rapidly and constantly evolving space of clinical importance to pediatric sleep providers and their patients. Our review provides clinicians with an up-to-date assessment of relevant issues about standard polysomnographic measurements and highlights potentially valuable insights to be found with more advanced spectral and autonomic analysis. Home sleep apnea testing in children remains a clinically prescient need, but validation studies have yielded mixed results. Furthermore, we caution readers to examine validation studies with a firm understanding of diagnostic concordance versus simple correlation. In the consumer space, there has been an explosion of devices for both sleep measurement and intervention, and there is exciting potential for these new tools.

CLINICS CARE POINTS

- Attention to technical issues related to polysomnographic signal acquisition aids in accurate sleep study interpretation.
- EEG spectral analysis or pulse-wave analysis may reveal important information regarding sleep disruption not captured by traditional sleep staging.
- Home sleep testing for pediatric OSA is not yet standard of care but remains an active area of research.

- Readers are directed to #SleepTechnology on the AASM website as an excellent up-to-date resource on consumer sleep technology.
- When evaluating potential novel sleep measurement approaches, clinicians should be mindful of accurately interpreting diagnostic agreement statistics to apply these technologies appropriately.

DISCLOSURE

The authors have no relevant financial relationships or conflicts of interest to disclose.

REFERENCES

1. Baughn JM, Lechner HG, Herold DL, et al. Enhancing the patient and family experience during pediatric sleep studies. J Clin Sleep Med 2020;16(7):1037–43.
2. Borbély AA, Baumann F, Brandeis D, et al. Sleep deprivation: effect on sleep stages and EEG power density in man. Electroencephalogr Clin Neurophysiol 1981;51(5):483–95.
3. Campbell IG, Feinberg I. Homeostatic sleep response to naps is similar in normal elderly and young adults. Neurobiol Aging 2005;26(1):135–44.
4. Merica H, Blois R, Gaillard JM. Spectral characteristics of sleep EEG in chronic insomnia. Eur J Neurosci 1998;10(5):1826–34.
5. Keshavan MS, Reynolds CF 3rd, Miewald MJ, et al. Delta sleep deficits in schizophrenia: evidence from automated analyses of sleep data. Arch Gen Psychiatry 1998;55(5):443–8.
6. Bandla HP, Gozal D. Dynamic changes in EEG spectra during obstructive apnea in children. Pediatr Pulmonol 2000;29(5):359–65.
7. Gutiérrez-Tobal GC, Gomez-Pilar J, Kheirandish-Gozal L, et al. Pediatric sleep apnea: the overnight Electroencephalogram as a phenotypic biomarker. Front Neurosci 2021;15:644697.
8. Catcheside PG, Chiong SC, Mercer J, et al. Noninvasive cardiovascular markers of acoustically induced arousal from non-rapid-eye-movement sleep. Sleep 2002;25(7):797–804.
9. Davies RJ, Belt PJ, Roberts SJ, et al. Arterial blood pressure responses to graded transient arousal from sleep in normal humans. J Appl Phys 1993;74(3):1123–30.
10. Guilleminault C, Connolly S, Winkle R, et al. Cyclical variation of the heart rate in sleep apnoea syndrome. Mechanisms, and usefulness of 24 h electrocardiography as a screening technique. Lancet 1984;1(8369):126–31.
11. Tauman R, O'Brien LM, Mast BT, et al. Peripheral arterial tonometry events and

electroencephalographic arousals in children. Sleep 2004;27(3):502–6.

12. Pépin JL, Delavie N, Pin I, et al. Pulse transit time improves detection of sleep respiratory events and microarousals in children. Chest 2005;127(3):722–30.

13. Pitson D, Chhina N, Knijn S, et al. Changes in pulse transit time and pulse rate as markers of arousal from sleep in normal subjects. Clin Sci (Lond) 1994;87(2):269–73.

14. Goh DY, Galster P, Marcus CL. Sleep architecture and respiratory disturbances in children with obstructive sleep apnea. Am J Respir Crit Care Med 2000;162(2 Pt 1):682–6.

15. O'Brien LM, Gozal D. Potential usefulness of noninvasive autonomic monitoring in recognition of arousals in normal healthy children. J Clin Sleep Med 2007;3(1):41–7.

16. Al-Shawwa B, Cruz J, Ehsan Z, et al. The challenges in scoring hypopneas in children: is pulse wave amplitude drop the answer? Sleep Med 2021;81: 336–40.

17. Massie F, Van Pee B, Bergmann J. Correlations between home sleep apnea tests and polysomnography outcomes do not fully reflect the diagnostic accuracy of these tests. J Clin Sleep Med 2022; 18(3):871–6.

18. Kirk V, Baughn J, D'Andrea L, et al. American Academy of sleep medicine position paper for the use of a home sleep apnea test for the diagnosis of OSA in children. J Clin Sleep Med 2017;13(10):1199–203.

19. Masoud AI, Patwari PP, Adavadkar PA, et al. Validation of the MediByte portable monitor for the diagnosis of sleep apnea in pediatric patients. J Clin Sleep Med 2019;15(5):733–42.

20. Vézina K, Mariasine J, Young R, et al. Cardiorespiratory monitoring data during sleep in healthy Canadian infants. Ann Am Thorac Soc 2020;17(10): 1238–46.

21. Westenberg JN, Petrof BJ, Noel F, et al. Validation of home portable monitoring for the diagnosis of sleep-disordered breathing in adolescents and adults with neuromuscular disorders. J Clin Sleep Med 2021; 17(8):1579–90.

22. Cheung TW, Lam DS, Chan PC, et al. Comparing respiratory polygraphy with pulse transit time analysis versus overnight polysomnography in the diagnosis of obstructive sleep apnoea in children. Sleep Med 2021;81:457–62.

23. Lildal TK, Bertelsen JB, Ovesen T. Feasibility of conducting type III home sleep apnoea test in children. Acta Otolaryngol 2021;141(7):707–13.

24. Revana A, Vecchio J, Guffey D, et al. Clinical application of home sleep apnea testing in children: a prospective pilot study. J Clin Sleep Med 2022; 18(2):533–40.

25. Green A, Nagel N, Kemer L, et al. Comparing in-lab full polysomnography for diagnosing sleep apnea in children to home sleep apnea tests (HSAT) with an online video attending technician. Sleep Biol Rhythms 2022;1–5.

26. Griffiths A, Mukushi A, Adams AM. Telehealth-supported level 2 pediatric home polysomnography. J Clin Sleep Med 2022. https://doi.org/10.5664/ jcsm.9982.

27. Wu CR, Tu YK, Chuang LP, et al. Diagnostic meta-analysis of the Pediatric Sleep Questionnaire, OSA-18, and pulse oximetry in detecting pediatric obstructive sleep apnea syndrome. Sleep Med Rev 2020;54:101355. https://doi.org/10.1016/j.smrv. 2020.101355.

28. Galway NC, Maxwell B, Shields M, et al. Use of oximetry to screen for paediatric obstructive sleep apnoea: is one night enough and is 6 hours too much? Arch Dis Child 2021;106(1):58–61.

29. Hoppenbrouwer XLR, Rollinson AU, Dunsmuir D, et al. Night to night variability of pulse oximetry features in children at home and at the hospital. Physiol Meas 2021;(10):42. https://doi.org/10.1088/1361-6579/ac278e.

30. Su M, Yu C, Zhang Y, et al. [Clinical value of portable sleep testing in children with obstructive sleep apnea syndrome]. Zhonghua Er Ke Za Zhi 2015; 53(11):845–9.

31. Serra A, Cocuzza S, Maiolino L, et al. The watch-pat in pediatrics sleep disordered breathing: pilot study on children with negative nocturnal pulse oximetry. Int J Pediatr Otorhinolaryngol 2017;97:245–50.

32. Tanphaichitr A, Thianboonsong A, Banhiran W, et al. Watch peripheral arterial tonometry in the diagnosis of pediatric obstructive sleep apnea. Otolaryngol Head Neck Surg 2018;159(1):166–72.

33. Norman MB, Pithers SM, Teng AY, et al. Validation of the Sonomat against PSG and Quantitative measurement of partial upper airway obstruction in children with sleep-disordered breathing. Sleep 2017; 40(3). https://doi.org/10.1093/sleep/zsx017.

34. Norman MB, Harrison HC, Waters KA, et al. Snoring and stertor are associated with more sleep disturbance than apneas and hypopneas in pediatric SDB. Sleep Breath 2019;23(4):1245–54.

35. D'Souza B, Norman M, Sullivan CE, et al. TcCO(2) changes correlate with partial obstruction in children suspected of sleep disordered breathing. Pediatr Pulmonol 2020;55(10):2773–81.

36. Norman MB, Harrison HC, Sullivan CE, et al. Measurement of snoring and stertor using the Sonomat to assess effectiveness of upper airway surgery in children. J Clin Sleep Med 2022. https://doi.org/10. 5664/jcsm.9946.

37. Khosla S, Deak MC, Gault D, et al. Consumer sleep technology: an American Academy of sleep medicine position statement. J Clin Sleep Med : JCSM : official publication of the American Academy of Sleep Medicine 2018;14(5):877–80.

38. Lee XK, Chee NIYN, Ong JL, et al. Validation of a consumer sleep wearable device with actigraphy and polysomnography in adolescents across sleep opportunity manipulations. J Clin Sleep Med 2019; 15(09):1337–46.

39. de Zambotti M, Goldstone A, Claudatos S, et al. A validation study of Fitbit Charge 2™ compared with polysomnography in adults. Chronobiol Int 2018;35(4):465–76.

40. Cook JD, Prairie ML, Plante DT. Ability of the multi-sensory Jawbone UP3 to quantify and classify sleep in patients with suspected central disorders of hypersomnolence: a comparison against polysomnography and actigraphy. J Clin Sleep Med 2018; 14(05):841–8.

41. Pesonen A-K, Kuula L. The validity of a new consumer-targeted wrist device in sleep measurement: an overnight comparison against polysomnography in children and adolescents. J Clin Sleep Med 2018;14(04):585–91.

42. Berryhill S, Morton CJ, Dean A, et al. Effect of wearables on sleep in healthy individuals: a randomized crossover trial and validation study. J Clin Sleep Med 2020;16(5):775–83.

43. van Kooten JAMC, Jacobse STW, Heymans MW, et al. A meta-analysis of accelerometer sleep outcomes in healthy children based on the Sadeh algorithm: the influence of child and device characteristics. Sleep 2020;44(4). https://doi.org/10.1093/sleep/zsaa231.

44. Burkart S, Beets MW, Armstrong B, et al. Comparison of multichannel and single-channel wrist-based devices with polysomnography to measure sleep in children and adolescents. J Clin Sleep Med 2021; 17(4):645–52.

45. Kirszenblat R, Edouard P. Validation of the withings ScanWatch as a wrist-worn reflective pulse oximeter: prospective interventional clinical study. J Med Internet Res 2021;23(4):e27503.

46. Gu W, Leung L, Kwok KC, et al. Belun Ring Platform: a novel home sleep apnea testing system for assessment of obstructive sleep apnea. J Clin Sleep Med 2020;16(9):1611–7.

47. Massie F, Almeida DMd, Dreesen P, et al. An evaluation of the NightOwl home sleep apnea testing system. J Clin Sleep Med 2018;14(10):1791–6.

48. de Zambotti M, Rosas L, Colrain IM, et al. The sleep of the ring: comparison of the ŌURA sleep tracker against polysomnography. Behav Sleep Med 2019; 17(2):124–36.

49. Ashry HSA, Hilmisson H, Ni Y, et al. Automated apnea–hypopnea index from oximetry and spectral analysis of cardiopulmonary coupling. Annals of the American Thoracic Society 2021;18(5):876–83.

50. Hilmisson H, Berman S, Magnusdottir S. Sleep apnea diagnosis in children using software-generated apnea-hypopnea index (AHI) derived from data recorded with a single photoplethysmogram sensor (PPG). Sleep Breath 2020;24(4):1739–49.

51. Thomas RJ, Wood C, Bianchi MT. Cardiopulmonary coupling spectrogram as an ambulatory clinical biomarker of sleep stability and quality in health, sleep apnea, and insomnia. Sleep 2017;41(2). https://doi.org/10.1093/sleep/zsx196.

52. Thomas RJ, Kim H, Maillard P, et al. Digital sleep measures and white matter health in the Framingham Heart Study. Exploration of Medicine 2021; 2(3):253–67.

53. Bonafide CP, Localio AR, Ferro DF, et al. Accuracy of pulse oximetry-based home baby monitors. JAMA 2018;320(7):717–9.

54. Malik A, Ehsan Z. Media review: the owlet Smart Sock—a "must have" for the baby registry? J Clin Sleep Med 2020;16(5):839–40.

55. Martinot JB, Cuthbert V, Le-Dong NN, et al. Clinical validation of a mandibular movement signal based system for the diagnosis of pediatric sleep apnea. Pediatr Pulmonol 2021. https://doi.org/10.1002/ppul.25320.

56. Tuominen J, Peltola K, Saaresranta T, et al. Sleep parameter assessment accuracy of a consumer home sleep monitoring Ballistocardiograph Beddit sleep tracker: a validation study. J Clin Sleep Med 2019;15(3):483–7.

57. Lauteslager T, Kampakis S, Williams AJ, et al. Performance evaluation of the Circadia Contactless breathing monitor and sleep analysis algorithm for sleep stage classification. Annu Int Conf IEEE Eng Med Biol Soc 2020;2020:5150–3.

58. Schade MM, Bauer CE, Murray BR, et al. Sleep validity of a non-contact Bedside movement and respiration-Sensing device. J Clin Sleep Med 2019; 15(07):1051–61.

59. Toften S, Pallesen S, Hrozanova M, et al. Validation of sleep stage classification using non-contact radar technology and machine learning (Somnofy®). Sleep Med 2020;75:54–61.

60. Arnal PJ, Thorey V, Debellemaniere E, et al. The Dreem Headband compared to polysomnography for electroencephalographic signal acquisition and sleep staging. Sleep 2020;43(11). https://doi.org/10.1093/sleep/zsaa097.

61. Levendowski DJ, Ferini-Strambi L, Gamaldo C, et al. The accuracy, night-to-night variability, and stability of frontopolar sleep Electroencephalography Biomarkers. J Clin Sleep Med 2017;13(06): 791–803.

62. Finan PH, Richards JM, Gamaldo CE, et al. Validation of a wireless, Self-application, ambulatory electroencephalographic sleep monitoring device in healthy volunteers. J Clin Sleep Med 2016;12(11): 1443–51.

63. Kram JA, Woidtke RV, Klein KB, et al. Evaluation of continuous negative external pressure (cNEP) for

the treatment of obstructive sleep apnea: a pilot study. J Clin Sleep Med 2017;13(08):1009–12.

64. Baptista PM, Martínez Ruiz de Apodaca P, Carrasco M, et al. Daytime neuromuscular electrical therapy of tongue muscles in improving snoring in individuals with primary snoring and mild obstructive sleep apnea. J Clin Med 2021;10(9):1883.

65. Cheng C-Y, Chen C-C, Lo M-T, et al. Evaluation of efficacy and safety of intraoral negative air pressure device in adults with obstructive sleep apnea in Taiwan. Sleep Med 2021;81:163–8.

66. Roth T, Mayleben D, Feldman N, et al. A novel forehead temperature-regulating device for insomnia: a randomized clinical trial. Sleep 2018;41(5). https://doi.org/10.1093/sleep/zsy045.

67. Comtet H, Geoffroy PA, Kobayashi Frisk M, et al. Light therapy with boxes or glasses to counteract effects of acute sleep deprivation. Sci Rep 2019;9(1):18073.

68. Langevin RH, Laurent A, Sauvé Y. Évaluation préliminaire de l'efficacité de la Luminette® chez des adolescents atteints du syndrome de retard de phase du sommeil (SRPS) : essai randomisé en simple insu et contrôlé par placebo. Médecine du Sommeil. 2014;11(2):91–7.

69. Ftouni S, Sletten TL, Howard M, et al. Objective and subjective measures of sleepiness, and their associations with on-road driving events in shift workers. J Sleep Res 2013;22(1):58–69.

70. Gabel V, Miglis M, Zeitzer JM. Effect of artificial dawn light on cardiovascular function, alertness, and balance in middle-aged and older adults. Sleep 2020;43(10). https://doi.org/10.1093/sleep/zsaa082.

71. Giménez MC, Hessels M, van de Werken M, et al. Effects of artificial dawn on subjective ratings of sleep inertia and dim light melatonin onset. Chronobiol Int 2010;27(6):1219–41.

72. Van De Werken M, Giménez MC, De Vries B, et al. Effects of artificial dawn on sleep inertia, skin temperature, and the awakening cortisol response. J Sleep Res 2010;19(3):425–35.

73. Schoen S, Man S, Spiro C. A sleep intervention for children with autism spectrum disorder: a pilot study. Open Journal of Occupational Therapy 2017. https://doi.org/10.15453/2168-6408.1293.

74. Rabin D, Siegle G. Toward Emotion prosthetics: Emotion regulation through wearable vibroacoustic stimulation. Biol Psychiatr 2018;83(9):S380–1.

75. Levendowski DJ, Seagraves S, Popovic D, et al. Assessment of a neck-based treatment and monitoring device for positional obstructive sleep apnea. J Clin Sleep Med 2014;10(08):863–71.

76. Berry RB, Uhles ML, Abaluck BK, et al. NightBalance sleep position treatment device versus auto-adjusting positive airway pressure for treatment of positional obstructive sleep apnea. J Clin Sleep Med 2019;15(07):947–56.

77. Ong JL, Patanaik A, Chee NIYN, et al. Auditory stimulation of sleep slow oscillations modulates subsequent memory encoding through altered hippocampal function. Sleep 2018;41(5). https://doi.org/10.1093/sleep/zsy031.

78. Mitchell UH, Hilton SC, Hunsaker E, et al. Decreased Symptoms without augmented skin blood flow in subjects with RLS/WED after vibration treatment. J Clin Sleep Med 2016;12(7):947–52.

79. Lack L, Scott H, Micic G, et al. Intensive sleep Retraining: from Bench to Bedside. Brain Sci 2017;7(4):33.

80. Hostler JM, Sheikh KL, Andrada TF, et al. A mobile, web-based system can improve positive airway pressure adherence. J Sleep Res 2017;26(2):139–46.

81. Malhotra A, Crocker ME, Willes L, et al. Patient Engagement using new technology to improve adherence to positive airway pressure therapy: a retrospective analysis. Chest 2018;153(4):843–50.

82. Nagare R, Plitnick B, Figueiro M. Does the iPad Night Shift mode reduce melatonin suppression? Light Res Technol 2019;51(3):373–83.

83. Narayan S, Shivdare P, Niranjan T, et al. Noncontact identification of sleep-disturbed breathing from smartphone-recorded sounds validated by polysomnography. Sleep Breath 2019;23(1):269–79.

84. Chaudhry BM. Sleeping with an android. mHealth 2017;3(2).

85. Akbar F, Weber I. #Sleep_as_Android: Feasibility of Using Sleep Logs on Twitter for Sleep Studies. 2016:227-233.

86. Patel P, Kim JY, Brooks LJ. Accuracy of a smartphone application in estimating sleep in children. Sleep Breath 2017;21(2):505–11.

87. Ritterband LM, Thorndike FP, Ingersoll KS, et al. Effect of a web-based cognitive behavior therapy for insomnia intervention with 1-year follow-up: a randomized clinical trial. JAMA Psychiatr 2017;74(1):68–75.

88. Christensen H, Batterham PJ, Gosling JA, et al. Effectiveness of an online insomnia program (SHUTi) for prevention of depressive episodes (the GoodNight Study): a randomised controlled trial. Lancet Psychiatr 2016;3(4):333–41.

Sleep and Mental Health Problems in Children and Adolescents

Isabel Morales-Muñoz, PhD[a],*, Alice M. Gregory, PhD[b]

KEYWORDS

• Sleep • Mental health • Children • Adolescent • Narrative review

KEY POINTS

- There are complex and bidirectional associations between sleep and mental health.
- In the last decade, there has been an increase in longitudinal studies focusing on sleep and mental health.
- Further research should focus on sleep and mental health in early childhood.
- There is a need to further investigate the mechanisms underlying the associations between sleep and different aspects of mental health.

INTRODUCTION

Sleep disturbances are often observed in children and adolescents.[1] For example, a recent study found that sleep-related difficulties were reported by parents in 22.6% of children and 20.0% of adolescents.[2] Similarly, many youths develop mental disorders in childhood and adolescence.[3] Childhood and adolescence are key periods in which to investigate mental health, as more than half of mental disorders start during these stages of life, and many persist throughout adulthood.[4] The worldwide prevalence of presenting with any mental disorder at some point during childhood or adolescence was estimated by one meta-analysis to be approximately 13%.[3]

Not only are sleep difficulties and mental health problems common but they go hand-in-hand. Although traditionally, sleep problems have been considered a secondary symptom of psychiatric conditions,[5] it is now clear that they warrant independent consideration and that there is a complex and bidirectional association between sleep and mental health.[6] Furthermore, there is increasing literature suggesting that sleep disturbances occur before the development of mental disorders.[7]

Previous reviews have described the links between sleep and mental health extensively.[8,9] With this in mind, this review focuses predominantly on research studies on this topic published during the last decade. Here, we focus largely on symptoms of mental disorders listed in the most recent edition of the Diagnostic and Statistical Manual of Mental Disorders (DSM-5).[10] More specifically, we focus on sleep in relation to neurodevelopmental disorders (ie, autism spectrum disorder [ASD] and attention-deficit hyperactivity disorder [ADHD]), Schizophrenia spectrum and other psychotic disorders, Bipolar disorders (BDs), Depressive disorders, Anxiety disorders, and Disruptive, impulse-control, and conduct disorders, as these are among the most common and/or pervasive mental disorders experienced by young people. Next, we discuss possible

a Institute for Mental Health, School of Psychology, University of Birmingham, 52 Pritchatts Road, Birmingham B15 2SA, UK; b Department of Psychology, Goldsmiths, University of London, Whitehead Building, New Cross, London SE14 6NW, United Kingdom
* Corresponding author. Institute for Mental Health, School of Psychology, University of Birmingham, 52 Pritchatts Road, Birmingham B15 2SA, UK.
E-mail address: I.Morales-Munoz@bham.ac.uk

Sleep Med Clin 18 (2023) 245–254
https://doi.org/10.1016/j.jsmc.2023.01.006
1556-407X/23/© 2023 Elsevier Inc. All rights reserved.

mechanisms underlying these associations. Finally, we flag possible lines of future enquiry.

SLEEP AND MENTAL HEALTH IN CHILDHOOD AND ADOLESCENCE
Sleep and Neurodevelopmental Disorders

Sleep disturbances are extremely prevalent in children with neurodevelopmental disorders.[11] In children with ASD, sleep problems are very common.[12] According to a review, some examples of sleep problems in these children include prolonged sleep latency, decreased sleep efficiency, reduced total sleep time, increased waking after sleep-onset, bedtime resistance, and daytime sleepiness.[13] Importantly, the temporal nature of the association between sleep problems and ASD is unclear because longitudinal studies are lacking, and the existing findings are contradictory. Some authors suggest that sleep problems do not precede autistic behavior but rather co-occur with autistic traits in early childhood,[14] whereas other research supports that sleep problems in early childhood (eg, reduced total sleep duration) are associated with ASD by age 11 years.[15]

There is growing evidence that ADHD is associated with poor sleep across the lifespan, including during childhood and adolescence.[16] Recent cross-sectional studies have described a wide range of sleep problems in children and adolescents with ADHD. Common sleep complaints reported by parents with children with ADHD include insomnia, excessive daytime sleepiness, and variability in sleep schedule,[17] in addition to greater sleep onset delay, sleep anxiety, night awakenings, and daytime sleepiness,[18] or problems falling asleep and parasomnias.[19] Parent-reported sleep problems in preschoolers with ADHD include delayed bedtime, increased sleep onset latency, and absence of naps.[20] Other cross-sectional studies have used objective sleep measures to investigate the sleep patterns in children and adolescents with ADHD. For example, in a meta-analysis investigating the use of actigraphy in children with ADHD, the results showed altered sleep onset latency and sleep efficiency in ADHD, whereas there was no evidence for differences in terms of sleep duration or wakefulness periods.[21] In preschoolers, those with ADHD as compared with age-matched typically developing preschool children, show increased motor activity during sleep and night-to-night variability for sleep duration,[22] whereas in toddlers early signs of ADHD are associated with irregular sleep patterns.[23] In adolescents, having ADHD is associated with shorter actigraphy-measured sleep duration.[24]

In recent years, there has been increased interest in longitudinal studies to investigate the prospective associations between sleep and ADHD. Although most of these longitudinal studies have investigated whether sleep problems precede subsequent ADHD, there is also some evidence to suggest that ADHD precedes sleep problems. For example, one study found that children with ADHD report poorer sleep quality in young adulthood, but only if their ADHD persists into adulthood.[25] The converse (ie, sleep problems precede ADHD) has also attracted research attention and existing evidence supports the idea that sleep problems in early childhood precedes ADHD. For example, parent-reported short sleep duration in early childhood is associated with ADHD in middle childhood.[26] Furthermore, shorter sleep duration and sleep disturbances in early childhood predate the typical age of clinical ADHD diagnosis,[27] and have been associated with inattention and hyperactivity at 5 years.[28] These prospective associations continue into adolescence, with recent evidence suggesting that several sleep problems in early childhood, including insomnia and frequent snoring,[29] as well as difficulty going to sleep, nightmares, and restless sleep,[30] predict ADHD in adolescence.

Sleep and Schizophrenia Spectrum and Other Psychotic Disorders

Psychotic disorders and schizophrenia are usually first diagnosed between 15 and 35 year old.[31] Therefore, this section will focus on psychotic symptoms that are more likely to be present in pediatric populations.

Cross-sectionally, there is evidence supporting the associations between psychotic experiences and sleep problems in pediatric populations. So far, there is scarce research focusing on children but existing research highlights that psychotic experiences in children associate with mother-reported nightmares, but not with actigraphic sleep measures.[32] Most of the cross-sectional research on the topic has been conducted in adolescence, and the existing research indicates that adolescents at ultra-high-risk for psychosis (UHR) display increased sleep onset latency and greater sleep disturbances,[33] in addition to greater wakefulness after sleep onset.[34] At the population level, existing evidence indicates that insomnia and excessive daytime sleepiness are associated with psychotic experiences in adolescents,[35] and that adolescents with long and short sleep duration are at higher risk of experiencing psychotic symptoms.[36]

Longitudinally, existing studies show that parent-reported nightmares across childhood are linked to self-reported psychotic experiences in early[37] and late adolescence.[38] Furthermore, parent-reported behavioral sleep problems in early childhood precede self-reported psychotic experiences in early adolescence.[39] Longitudinal studies using actigraphy show that several objective measures of sleep predict the longitudinal course of psychotic symptoms over 12 months in adolescents with UHR,[40] and that circadian disruptions also predict the severity of psychotic symptoms at 1-year follow-up among adolescents with UHR.[41]

Sleep and Bipolar Disorder

Sleep disturbance is a core symptom of BD.[42] The diagnostic criteria indicate that during manic episodes there may be a reduced need for sleep and during episodes of depression, insomnia or hypersomnia can be frequently experienced.[10] However, research on sleep disturbances in youth with BD is still scarce, partly due to controversy around the diagnosis of BD in children and adolescents.

Existing cross-sectional studies indicate that several sleep disturbances are associated with BD in children and adolescents.[43] Furthermore, greater sleep disturbances have been reported in unaffected child and adolescent offspring of bipolar parents as compared with controls.[44] When considering different symptoms of BD, longer time in bed and higher prevalence of nocturnal enuresis seem during depressive compared with manic episodes, whereas unrestful sleep is more common during manic episodes.[45] When comparing BD type I and BD not otherwise specified, there are no differences in the frequency of sleep symptoms.[46]

Longitudinal evidence suggests that sleep disturbances may predict BD. For example, sleep impairments were associated with mania and depression severity across a 2-year follow-up in adolescence.[47] When considering different aspects of sleep, one study found that a greater number of awakenings and longer time awake during the weekend predicted greater depression symptoms in adolescents with BD.[48] Furthermore, trouble falling asleep and early morning awakenings were also associated with subsequent BD.[49]

Sleep and Depressive Disorders

Sleep difficulties are among the core symptoms for the diagnostic criteria for depression,[50] and of all the mental disorders associated with insomnia, the link with depression is the most robust.[51] This

is not only true for adults, but increasing evidence supports the central role of sleep in childhood and adolescent depression. For example, insomnia is the most common residual symptom among depressed youth.[52]

Cross-sectionally, short sleep as compared with that of appropriate duration, has been associated with increased depressive symptoms in adolescents.[53] Shorter sleep duration and time in bed, as well as longer sleep latency and wake after sleep onset have also been reported in depressed adolescents, and particularly in boys.[54] Furthermore, one study found that participants with fewest depressive symptoms presented moderate sleep timing, shorter sleep-onset latencies, and fewer arousals as compared with those with more depressive symptoms.[55]

During the last decade, the number of longitudinal studies on sleep and depression in children and adolescents has increased dramatically. Some of these studies have considered the bidirectional association between sleep and depression in adolescence. For example, one study reported that sleep deprivation predicted both symptoms of depression and DSM-IV major depression at follow-up, whereas major depression, but not depression symptoms predicted sleep deprivation.[56] Another study reported that insomnia increased the subsequent risk for major depression and major depression increased the risk for subsequent insomnia.[57] Previous longitudinal research also suggests that between 9 and 16 years, sleep problems predict later depression symptoms, and in turn, depression predicts sleep problems.[58] Finally, in a recent study, maternal-reported short sleep duration and frequent night waking at 1.5 years predicted maternal-reported depressive symptoms at 8 years, and in turn maternal-reported depressive symptoms at 1.5 years predicted the onset of later maternal-reported short sleep duration.[59]

Some other longitudinal studies have focused on sleep problems as a precursor of depression. For example, cumulative sleep deprivation was found to increase depression at follow-up in females, but not males, during adolescence.[60] Further, sleep duration <8h and ≥ 9h on weekdays; and <8 h and ≥ 12 h on weekends have all been associated with depressive symptoms in adolescents over 2 years.[61] Further, greater sleep disturbances (as compared with other mental disorders) were stronger predictors of depression in early adolescence at 1-year follow-up.[62] Finally, sleep apnea has received recent attention, with evidence suggesting that childhood apnea is a risk for subsequent depressive disorders.[63]

Sleep and Anxiety Disorders

Sleep problems are common in children and adolescents with anxiety disorders with one study reporting that more than 80% of youth with anxiety disorders experience at least one sleep-related problem, and 55% experience three or more.[64]

Cross-sectionally, recent research conducted in children indicates that generalized anxiety disorder symptoms (GAD) are associated with increased parental-reported sleep concerns in school-aged children.[65] Furthermore, late bedtime and short sleep duration are associated with children's anxious behavior.[66] In adolescence, reduced hours of sleep have been associated with anxiety symptoms,[67] and adolescents with obstructive sleep apnea report more severe anxiety symptoms.[68]

Longitudinally, the bidirectional associations between sleep and anxiety in young populations have been examined. Existing research supports the role of sleep problems as risk factors for anxiety symptoms in adolescence, with less evidence for the reverse. For example, a recent study found that poor sleep, especially during early and mid-adolescence precedes anxiety symptoms,[69] but not the other way around. Furthermore, reduced sleep quantity increases risk for anxiety, but anxiety does not increase the risk for decreased sleep duration among adolescents.[70] Other research suggests that the bidirectionality may vary by subtypes of sleep problems and anxiety symptoms. For example, short sleep duration predicted symptoms of panic disorder, GAD, and school phobia; and was predicted by GAD in adolescents.[71]

A further longitudinal study found that a range of sleep variables at age 15 predicted the severity and the diagnoses of anxiety at age 17, 21, and 24 years.[72] It has also been reported that sleep problems at 2 years are significantly associated with anxiety at 8 years,[73] and infants with persistent severe sleep problems during the first postnatal year have an increased risk for anxiety at age 10.[74]

Sleep and composites of internalizing problems in childhood and adolescence

When investigating anxiety and depression in young people, many studies refer to internalizing problems, which include items about both anxiety and depression.

Most recent studies on the topic have investigated longitudinal associations. Some have investigated the potential bidirectionality of these associations, but the results are inconsistent. For example, one study reported that sleep problems predicted changes in internalizing problems over time in young adolescents, but not the other way around.[75] In addition, another study conducted on school-aged children found that sleep problems preceded later internalizing difficulties but not vice versa.[76] However, a further study found that mother-reported sleep problems at 6 years were predictive of self-reported internalizing problems at 11.5 years, and at 6 years, teacher-reported and mother-rated internalizing problems were related to sleep problems at 11.5 years.[77] A study of toddlers also found reciprocal associations between trouble getting to sleep and internalizing problems.[78]

Other longitudinal studies have focused on the role of sleep as a precursor of internalizing problems across childhood and adolescence. For example, in early childhood, shorter sleep and poorer sleep quality in infancy was related to internalizing symptoms in toddlers.[79] Further, later bedtimes and less total sleep in infancy were associated with internalizing issues in toddlers,[80] and short sleep duration and frequent nocturnal awakenings in children at 18 months related to internalizing problems at 5 years.[81] In adolescents, persistent sleeping difficulties in females aged 12/13 years predicted internalizing problems at 14/15 years.[82]

Sleep and Disruptive, Impulse-Control, and Conduct Disorders

Cross-sectionally, existing evidence suggests that children with conduct disorder report more sleep problems than control children.[83] Furthermore, shorter nighttime sleep duration in preschool children has been associated with higher overactivity, anger, aggression, impulsivity, and tantrums based on parental reports.[84] Associations have been also reported between obstructive sleep apnea and conduct disorder in children.[85]

There is also longitudinal evidence to support bidirectional associations between sleep problems and disruptive behavior during childhood, with greater sleep problems associated with later disruptive behavior and vice versa.[86] Other longitudinal studies have reported that childhood conduct problems are linked to subsequent sleep problems in adolescence.[87] Furthermore, the reverse has been investigated and existing research suggests that longer sleep duration and higher sleep efficiency are linked to fewer externalizing symptoms at 1-year follow-up in children.[88] Finally, early-life sleep-disordered breathing symptoms seem to have strong, persistent effects on subsequent disruptive behavior in childhood.[89]

POTENTIAL UNDERLYING MECHANISMS IN THE ASSOCIATIONS BETWEEN SLEEP AND MENTAL HEALTH

It is increasingly well-established that sleep is linked to mental health, but an understanding of the mechanisms underlying associations lags behind. A greater understanding of the mechanisms will enable us to design more targeted interventions in mental health. Current research points to biological, psychological, and social mechanisms, and suggests the presence of sequential, parallel, and interacting underlying risk factors.[90] Here, we present just a few of the mechanisms that have received the greatest research attention, including (i) the family environment; (ii) genetic factors; and (iii) brain mechanisms.

Family Environment

A young person's sleep must be considered within the family context.[91] Parenting practices are among the many familial factors that could be linked to poor sleep and mental health problems in youth. For example, adverse parenting styles (eg, low positivity and high negativity) have been found to be associated with low sleep quality, negative mood, daytime sleepiness, and anxiety/depression symptoms among adolescents,[92] whereas positive parenting behaviors seem to promote good sleep behaviors and consequently reduce the risk for problematic behaviors among adolescents.[93]

Family stress (eg, family conflict) also has an impact on sleep development and mental disorders in young people. Overall, the existing evidence suggests that family stress has been associated with both insomnia and internalizing symptoms in adolescents.[90] For example, one study reported that stressful family events were associated with depressive symptoms in adolescents, and that this relationship was strongest among those with lower sleep quality. Therefore, parenting practices and family stress are both contributors to the relationship between sleep and mental health problems in the pediatric population.

Genetic Factors

There is evidence from twin studies supporting the existence of a strong overlap between genetic influences on symptoms of sleep and mental disorders. For example, recent reviews highlight a role for genetic factors in the associations between sleep variables and other factors, including anxiety, depression, psychotic-like experience, or externalizing behaviors, among others.[94,95]

Furthermore, recent evidence from genome-wide association studies supports genetic overlap between sleep-related phenotypes and BD, depression, and schizophrenia.[96] However, other studies indicate that insomnia has the strongest genetic correlations with depression, anxiety, and ADHD, whereas the genetic correlations between insomnia with schizophrenia and BD are lower.[97] Further, recent research using polygenic risk scores suggests that greater genetic susceptibility to ADHD, major depressive disorder, and anxiety disorders may contribute to greater sleep problems among children.[98]

Brain Mechanisms

Among the potential brain mechanisms, the prefrontal cortex plays a critical role in the regulation of sleep[99] and the regulation of the affective systems.[100] A recent study reported that longer sleep duration in adolescents correlated with a higher volume of the orbitofrontal and prefrontal cortex.[101] Other studies indicate that the medial prefrontal cortex correlates with bedtime and wake-up times in adolescents,[102] and that adolescents with poorer sleep also show less recruitment of the dorsolateral prefrontal cortex during cognitive control.[103] So far, only two studies have examined the associations between sleep and prefrontal brain areas in children. In one of these studies, sleep duration contributed to neural alterations of prefrontal areas in male children.[104] The second study used a longitudinal cohort study, finding that more adverse sleep disturbances during childhood were associated with a thinner dorsolateral prefrontal cortex.[105]

Further, the role that the prefrontal cortex plays in mental health is well established. For example, dysfunction of the prefrontal cortex is a central feature of many psychiatric disorders.[106] Therefore, it could be hypothesized that prefrontal cortex functioning could help to explain the associations between sleep and mental disorders. Specific studies examining how exactly the prefrontal cortex might mediate these associations are required.

SUMMARY

In this narrative review, we present the most recent literature investigating the link between sleep and mental health problems in childhood and adolescence. In the last decade, there has been an increase in longitudinal studies, allowing more information about the potential bi-directionality of associations as well as hints about the potential causal role of sleep in the development of specific mental disorders. To date, more research focuses on adolescence as compared with early childhood and further research should focus on these early stages.

There are three areas that should be considered in future investigation. First, there should be further investigation of the mechanisms underlying the associations between sleep and mental health. Although we have presented here few candidate mechanisms, there are many more mechanisms that could help to account for the associations between sleep and mental health. Second, further research using large population-based cohort studies to investigate the impact of early childhood sleep problems on youth mental health is still needed. Although some studies have been published recently, further evidence on how sleep problems in early childhood can lead to the development of mental disorders are still needed. Finally, future studies should focus on the treatment of sleep difficulties to prevent or reduce mental health difficulties. This line of enquiry has proved fruitful,[107] but intervention studies focusing on childhood and adolescence are still very scarce.

CLINICS CARE POINTS

- Sleep problems are associated with a wide range of mental health problems in childhood and adolescence.
- Sleep and mental health problems in young people present a bi-directional relationship.
- There are number of potential mechanisms explaining the links between sleep and mental health in young people.

DISCLOSURE

The authors have no financial relationships relevant to this article to disclose.

REFERENCES

1. Kotagal S, Pianosi P. Sleep disorders in children and adolescents. BMJ 2006;332(7545):828–32.
2. Lewien C, Genuneit J, Meigen C, et al. Sleep-related difficulties in healthy children and adolescents. BMC Pediatr 2021;21(1):82.
3. Polanczyk GV, Salum GA, Sugaya LS, et al. Annual research review: a meta-analysis of the worldwide prevalence of mental disorders in children and adolescents. J Child Psychol Psychiatry 2015;56(3): 345–65.
4. Kim-Cohen J, Caspi A, Moffitt TE, et al. Prior juvenile diagnoses in adults with mental disorder: developmental follow-back of a prospective-longitudinal cohort. Arch Gen Psychiatry 2003; 60(7):709–17.
5. Harvey AG. INSOMNIA: symptom OR DIAGNOSIS? Clin Psychol Rev 2001;21(7):1037–59.
6. Alvaro PK, Roberts RM, Harris JK. A systematic review assessing bidirectionality between sleep disturbances, anxiety, and depression. Sleep 2013; 36(7):1059–68.
7. Baglioni C, Battagliese G, Feige B, et al. Insomnia as a predictor of depression: a meta-analytic evaluation of longitudinal epidemiological studies. J Affect Disord 2011;135(1–3):10–9.
8. Gregory AM, O'Connor TG. Sleep problems in childhood: a longitudinal study of developmental change and association with behavioral problems. J Am Acad Child Adolesc Psychiatry 2002;41(8): 964–71.
9. Gregory AM, Sadeh A. Annual Research Review: sleep problems in childhood psychiatric disorders – a review of the latest science. J Child Psychol Psychiatry 2016;57(3):296–317.
10. American Psychiatric Association. Diagnostic and statistical manual of mental disorders. 5th edition. Arlington, VA: American Psychiatric Association; 2013.
11. Robinson-Shelton A, Malow BA. Sleep disturbances in neurodevelopmental disorders. Curr Psychiatry Rep 2016;18(1):6.
12. Veatch OJ, Maxwell-Horn AC, Malow BA. Sleep in autism spectrum disorders. Curr sleep Med reports 2015;1(2):131–40.
13. Cohen S, Conduit R, Lockley SW, et al. The relationship between sleep and behavior in autism spectrum disorder (ASD): a review. J Neurodev Disord 2014;6(1):44.
14. Verhoeff ME, Blanken LME, Kocevska D, et al. The bidirectional association between sleep problems and autism spectrum disorder: a population-based cohort study. Mol Autism 2018;9:8.
15. Humphreys JS, Gringras P, Blair PS, et al. Sleep patterns in children with autistic spectrum disorders: a prospective cohort study. Arch Dis Child 2014;99(2):114–8.
16. Becker SP. ADHD and sleep: recent advances and future directions. Curr Opin Psychol 2020;34:50–6.
17. Craig SG, Weiss MD, Hudec KL, et al. The functional impact of sleep disorders in children with ADHD. J Atten Disord 2020;24(4):499–508.
18. Schneider HE, Lam JC, Mahone EM. Sleep disturbance and neuropsychological function in young children with ADHD. Child Neuropsychol 2016; 22(4):493–506.
19. Vélez-Galarraga R, Guillén-Grima F, Crespo-Eguílaz N, et al. Prevalence of sleep disorders

and their relationship with core symptoms of inattention and hyperactivity in children with attention-deficit/hyperactivity disorder. Eur J Paediatr Neurol 2016;20(6):925–37.

20. Cao H, Yan S, Gu C, et al. Prevalence of attention-deficit/hyperactivity disorder symptoms and their associations with sleep schedules and sleep-related problems among preschoolers in mainland China. BMC Pediatr 2018;18(1):70.

21. De Crescenzo F, Licchelli S, Ciabattini M, et al. The use of actigraphy in the monitoring of sleep and activity in ADHD: a meta-analysis. Sleep Med Rev 2016;26:9–20.

22. Melegari MG, Vittori E, Mallia L, et al. Actigraphic sleep pattern of preschoolers with ADHD. J Atten Disord 2020;24(4):611–24.

23. Bundgaard A-KF, Asmussen J, Pedersen NS, et al. Disturbed sleep and activity in toddlers with early signs of attention deficit hyperactivity disorder (ADHD). J Sleep Res 2018;27(5):e12686.

24. Becker SP, Langberg JM, Eadeh H-M, et al. Sleep and daytime sleepiness in adolescents with and without ADHD: differences across ratings, daily diary, and actigraphy. J Child Psychol Psychiatry 2019;60(9):1021–31.

25. Gregory AM, Agnew-Blais JC, Matthews T, et al. ADHD and sleep quality: longitudinal analyses from childhood to early adulthood in a twin cohort. J Clin child Adolesc Psychol 2017;46(2):284–94.

26. Tso W, Chan M, Ho FK, et al. Early sleep deprivation and attention-deficit/hyperactivity disorder. Pediatr Res 2019;85(4):449–55.

27. Scott N, Blair PS, Emond AM, et al. Sleep patterns in children with ADHD: a population-based cohort study from birth to 11 years. J Sleep Res 2013;22(2):121–8.

28. Huhdanpaa H, Morales-Munoz I, Aronen ET, et al. Sleep difficulties in infancy are associated with symptoms of inattention and hyperactivity at the age of 5 Years: a longitudinal study. J Dev Behav Pediatr 2019;40(6):432–40.

29. Liu X, Liu Z-Z, Liu B-P, et al. Associations between sleep problems and ADHD symptoms among adolescents: findings from the Shandong Adolescent Behavior and Health Cohort (SABHC). Sleep 2020;43(6):zsz294.

30. Carpena MX, Munhoz TN, Xavier MO, et al. The role of sleep duration and sleep problems during childhood in the development of ADHD in adolescence: findings from a population-based birth cohort. J Atten Disord 2020;24(4):590–600.

31. Solmi M, Radua J, Olivola M, et al. Age at onset of mental disorders worldwide: large-scale meta-analysis of 192 epidemiological studies. Mol Psychiatry 2021;27(1):281–95.

32. Koopman-Verhoeff ME, Bolhuis K, Cecil CAM, et al. During day and night: childhood psychotic experiences and objective and subjective sleep problems. Schizophr Res 2019;206:127–34.

33. Lunsford-Avery JR, Orr JM, Gupta T, et al. Sleep dysfunction and thalamic abnormalities in adolescents at ultra high-risk for psychosis. Schizophr Res 2013;151(1–3):148–53.

34. Mayeli A, LaGoy A, Donati FL, et al. Sleep abnormalities in individuals at clinical high risk for psychosis. J Psychiatr Res 2021;137:328–34.

35. Lee YJ, Cho S-J, Cho IH, et al. The relationship between psychotic-like experiences and sleep disturbances in adolescents. Sleep Med 2012;13(8):1021–7.

36. Morishima R, Yamasaki S, Ando S, et al. Long and short sleep duration and psychotic symptoms in adolescents: findings from a cross-sectional survey of 15 786 Japanese students. Psychiatry Res 2020;293:113440.

37. Fisher HL, Lereya ST, Thompson A, et al. Childhood parasomnias and psychotic experiences at age 12 years in a United Kingdom birth cohort. Sleep 2014;37(3):475–82.

38. Thompson A, Lereya ST, Lewis G, et al. Childhood sleep disturbance and risk of psychotic experiences at 18: UK birth cohort. Br J Psychiatry 2015;207(1):23–9.

39. Morales-Muñoz I, Broome MR, Marwaha S. Association of parent-reported sleep problems in early childhood with psychotic and borderline personality disorder symptoms in adolescence. JAMA Psychiatr 2020;77(12):1256–65.

40. Lunsford-Avery JR, LeBourgeois MK, Gupta T, et al. Actigraphic-measured sleep disturbance predicts increased positive symptoms in adolescents at ultra high-risk for psychosis: a longitudinal study. Schizophr Res 2015;164(1–3):15–20.

41. Lunsford-Avery JR, Gonçalves B da SB, Brietzke E, et al. Adolescents at clinical-high risk for psychosis: circadian rhythm disturbances predict worsened prognosis at 1-year follow-up. Schizophr Res 2017;189:37–42.

42. Ng TH, Chung K-F, Ho FY-Y, et al. Sleep-wake disturbance in interepisode bipolar disorder and high-risk individuals: a systematic review and meta-analysis. Sleep Med Rev 2015;20:46–58.

43. Comsa M, Anderson KN, Sharma A, et al. The relationship between sleep and depression and bipolar disorder in children and young people. BJPsych open 2022;8(1):e27.

44. Sebela A, Kolenic M, Farkova E, et al. Decreased need for sleep as an endophenotype of bipolar disorder: an actigraphy study. Chronobiol Int 2019;36(9):1227–39.

45. Lopes MC, Boarati MA, Fu -IL. Sleep and daytime complaints during manic and depressive episodes in children and adolescents with bipolar disorder. Front psychiatry 2019;10:1021.

46. Baroni A, Hernandez M, Grant MC, et al. Sleep disturbances in pediatric bipolar disorder: a comparison between bipolar I and bipolar NOS. Front psychiatry 2012;3:22.

47. Lunsford-Avery JR, Judd CM, Axelson DA, et al. Sleep impairment, mood symptoms, and psychosocial functioning in adolescent bipolar disorder. Psychiatry Res 2012;200(2–3):265–71.

48. Gershon A, Singh MK. Sleep in adolescents with bipolar I disorder: stability and relation to symptom change. J Clin child Adolesc Psychol 2017;46(2): 247–57.

49. Ritter PS, Höfler M, Wittchen H-U, et al. Disturbed sleep as risk factor for the subsequent onset of bipolar disorder–Data from a 10-year prospective-longitudinal study among adolescents and young adults. J Psychiatr Res 2015;68:76–82.

50. Tolentino JC, Schmidt SL. DSM-5 criteria and depression severity: implications for clinical practice. Front Psychiatry 2018;9:450.

51. Krystal AD. Psychiatric disorders and sleep. Neurol Clin 2012;30(4):1389–413.

52. March J, Silva S, Petrycki S, et al. Fluoxetine, cognitive-behavioral therapy, and their combination for adolescents with depression: treatment for Adolescents with Depression Study (TADS) randomized controlled trial. JAMA 2004;292(7):807–20.

53. Yeo SC, Jos AM, Erwin C, et al. Associations of sleep duration on school nights with self-rated health, overweight, and depression symptoms in adolescents: problems and possible solutions. Sleep Med 2019;60:96–108.

54. Sivertsen B, Harvey AG, Lundervold AJ, et al. Sleep problems and depression in adolescence: results from a large population-based study of Norwegian adolescents aged 16-18 years. Eur Child Adolesc Psychiatry 2014;23(8):681–9.

55. Shochat T, Barker DH, Sharkey KM, et al. An approach to understanding sleep and depressed mood in adolescents: person-centred sleep classification. J Sleep Res 2017;26(6):709–17.

56. Roberts RE, Duong HT. The prospective association between sleep deprivation and depression among adolescents. Sleep 2014;37(2):239–44. https://doi.org/10.5665/sleep.3388.

57. Roberts RE, Duong HT. Depression and insomnia among adolescents: a prospective perspective. J Affect Disord 2013;148(1):66–71.

58. Shanahan L, Copeland WE, Angold A, et al. Sleep problems predict and are predicted by generalized anxiety/depression and oppositional defiant disorder. J Am Acad Child Adolesc Psychiatry 2014; 53(5):550–8.

59. Sivertsen B, Harvey AG, Reichborn-Kjennerud T, et al. Sleep problems and depressive symptoms in toddlers and 8-year-old children: a longitudinal study. J Sleep Res 2021;30(1):e13150.

60. Conklin AI, Yao CA, Richardson CG. Chronic sleep deprivation and gender-specific risk of depression in adolescents: a prospective population-based study. BMC Publ Health 2018;18(1):724.

61. Liu B-P, Wang X-T, Liu Z-Z, et al. Depressive symptoms are associated with short and long sleep duration: a longitudinal study of Chinese adolescents. J Affect Disord 2020;263:267–73.

62. Goldstone A, Javitz HS, Claudatos SA, et al. Sleep disturbance predicts depression symptoms in early adolescence: initial findings from the adolescent brain cognitive development study. J Adolesc Health 2020;66(5):567–74.

63. Chang C-H, Chen S-J, Liu C-Y. Pediatric sleep apnea and depressive disorders risk: a population-based 15-year retrospective cohort study. PLoS One 2017; 12(7):e0181430.

64. Alfano CA, Ginsburg GS, Kingery JN. Sleep-related problems among children and adolescents with anxiety disorders. J Am Acad Child Adolesc Psychiatry 2007;46(2):224–32.

65. Fletcher FE, Conduit R, Foster-Owens MD, et al. The association between anxiety symptoms and sleep in school-aged children: a combined insight from the children's sleep habits questionnaire and actigraphy. Behav Sleep Med 2018;16(2):169–84.

66. Suda M, Nagamitsu S, Obara H, et al. Association between children's sleep patterns and problematic behaviors at age 5. Pediatr Int 2020;62(10): 1189–96.

67. Sarchiapone M, Mandelli L, Carli V, et al. Hours of sleep in adolescents and its association with anxiety, emotional concerns, and suicidal ideation. Sleep Med 2014;15(2):248–54.

68. Park K-M, Kim S-Y, Sung D, et al. The relationship between risk of obstructive sleep apnea and other sleep problems, depression, and anxiety in adolescents from a community sample. Psychiatry Res 2019;280:112504.

69. Narmandakh A, Roest AM, Jonge P de, et al. The bidirectional association between sleep problems and anxiety symptoms in adolescents: a TRAILS report. Sleep Med 2020;67:39–46.

70. Roberts RE, Duong HT. Is there an association between short sleep duration and adolescent anxiety disorders? Sleep Med 2017;30:82–7.

71. Geng F, Liu X, Liang Y, et al. Prospective associations between sleep problems and subtypes of anxiety symptoms among disaster-exposed adolescents. Sleep Med 2018;50:7–13.

72. Orchard F, Gregory AM, Gradisar M, et al. Self-reported sleep patterns and quality amongst adolescents: cross-sectional and prospective associations with anxiety and depression. J Child Psychol Psychiatry 2020;61(10):1126–37.

73. Uren J, Richdale AL, Cotton SM, et al. Sleep problems and anxiety from 2 to 8 years and the

influence of autistic traits: a longitudinal study. Eur Child Adolesc Psychiatry 2019;28(8):1117–27.

74. Cook F, Conway LJ, Giallo R, et al. Infant sleep and child mental health: a longitudinal investigation. Arch Dis Child 2020;105(7):655–60.

75. Pieters S, Burk WJ, Van der Vorst H, et al. Prospective relationships between sleep problems and substance use, internalizing and externalizing problems. J Youth Adolesc 2015;44(2):379–88.

76. Williamson AA, Mindell JA, Hiscock H, et al. Longitudinal sleep problem trajectories are associated with multiple impairments in child well-being. J Child Psychol Psychiatry 2020;61(10):1092–103.

77. Liu J, Glenn AL, Cui N, et al. Longitudinal bidirectional association between sleep and behavior problems at age 6 and 11 years. Sleep Med 2021;83:290–8.

78. Conway A, Miller AL, Modrek A. Testing reciprocal links between trouble getting to sleep and internalizing behavior problems, and bedtime resistance and externalizing behavior problems in toddlers. Child Psychiatry Hum Dev 2017;48(4):678–89.

79. Morales-Muñoz I, Lemola S, Saarenpää-Heikkilä O, et al. Parent-reported early sleep problems and internalising, externalising and dysregulation symptoms in toddlers. BMJ Paediatr open 2020;4(1):e000622.

80. Mindell JA, Leichman ES, DuMond C, et al. Sleep and social-emotional development in infants and toddlers. J Clin Child Adolesc Psychol 2017;46(2):236–46.

81. Sivertsen B, Harvey AG, Reichborn-Kjennerud T, et al. Later emotional and behavioral problems associated with sleep problems in toddlers: a longitudinal study. JAMA Pediatr 2015;169(6):575–82.

82. Nunes S, Campbell MK, Klar N, et al. Relationships between sleep and internalizing problems in early adolescence: results from Canadian national longitudinal survey of children and youth. J Psychosom Res 2020;139:110279.

83. Aronen ET, Lampenius T, Fontell T, et al. Sleep in children with disruptive behavioral disorders. Behav Sleep Med 2014;12(5):373–88.

84. Scharf RJ, Demmer RT, Silver EJ, et al. Nighttime sleep duration and externalizing behaviors of preschool children. J Dev Behav Pediatr 2013;34(6):384–91.

85. Constantin E, Low NCP, Dugas E, et al. Association between childhood sleep-disordered breathing and disruptive behavior disorders in childhood and adolescence. Behav Sleep Med 2015;13(6):442–54.

86. Quach JL, Nguyen CD, Williams KE, et al. Bidirectional associations between child sleep problems and internalizing and externalizing difficulties from preschool to early adolescence. JAMA Pediatr 2018;172(2):e174363.

87. Tomasiello M, Temcheff CE, Martin-Storey A, et al. Self and parent-reported sleep problems of adolescents with childhood conduct problems and co-morbid psychological problems. J Adolesc 2021;92:165–76.

88. Belanger M-E, Bernier A, Simard V, et al. Sleeping toward behavioral regulation: relations between sleep and externalizing symptoms in toddlers and preschoolers. J Clin Child Adolesc Psychol 2018;47(3):366–73.

89. Bonuck K, Freeman K, Chervin RD, et al. Sleep-disordered breathing in a population-based cohort: behavioral outcomes at 4 and 7 years. Pediatrics 2012;129(4):e857–65.

90. Blake MJ, Trinder JA, Allen NB. Mechanisms underlying the association between insomnia, anxiety, and depression in adolescence: implications for behavioral sleep interventions. Clin Psychol Rev 2018;63:25–40.

91. Dahl RE, El-Sheikh M. Considering sleep in a family context: introduction to the special issue. J Fam Psychol 2007;21(1):1–3.

92. Brand S, Gerber M, Hatzinger M, et al. Evidence for similarities between adolescents and parents in sleep patterns. Sleep Med 2009;10(10):1124–31.

93. Vazsonyi AT, Harris C, Terveer AM, et al. Parallel mediation effects by sleep on the parental warmth-problem behavior links: evidence from national probability samples of Georgian and Swiss adolescents. J Youth Adolesc 2015;44(2):331–45.

94. Madrid-Valero JJ, Rubio-Aparicio M, Gregory AM, et al. Twin studies of subjective sleep quality and sleep duration, and their behavioral correlates: systematic review and meta-analysis of heritability estimates. Neurosci Biobehav Rev 2020;109:78–89.

95. Lewis KJS, Gregory AM. Heritability of sleep and its disorders in childhood and adolescence. Curr Sleep Med Reports 2021;7(4):155–66.

96. O'Connell KS, Frei O, Bahrami S, et al. Characterizing the genetic overlap between psychiatric disorders and sleep-related phenotypes. Biol Psychiatry 2021;90(9):621–31.

97. Byrne EM. The relationship between insomnia and complex diseases—insights from genetic data. Genome Med 2019;11(1):57.

98. Ohi K, Ochi R, Noda Y, et al. Polygenic risk scores for major psychiatric and neurodevelopmental disorders contribute to sleep disturbance in childhood: adolescent Brain Cognitive Development (ABCD) Study. Transl Psychiatry 2021;11(1):187.

99. Horne JA. Human sleep, sleep loss and behaviour. Implications for the prefrontal cortex and psychiatric disorder. Br J Psychiatry 1993;162:413–9.

100. Dahl RE. The regulation of sleep and arousal: development and psychopathology. Dev Psychopathol 1996;8(1):3–27.

101. Cheng W, Rolls E, Gong W, et al. Sleep duration, brain structure, and psychiatric and cognitive problems in children. Mol Psychiatry 2021;26(8):3992–4003.

102. Urrila AS, Artiges E, Massicotte J, et al. Sleep habits, academic performance, and the adolescent brain structure. Sci Rep 2017;7:41678.

103. Telzer EH, Fuligni AJ, Lieberman MD, et al. The effects of poor quality sleep on brain function and risk taking in adolescence. Neuroimage 2013;71:275–83.

104. Reidy BL, Hamann S, Inman C, et al. Decreased sleep duration is associated with increased fMRI responses to emotional faces in children. Neuropsychologia 2016;84:54–62.

105. Kocevska D, Muetzel RL, Luik AI, et al. The developmental course of sleep disturbances across childhood relates to brain morphology at age 7: the generation R study. Sleep 2017;40(1). https://doi.org/10.1093/sleep/zsw022.

106. Gamo NJ, Arnsten AFT. Molecular modulation of prefrontal cortex: rational development of treatments for psychiatric disorders. Behav Neurosci 2011; 125(3):282–96.

107. Freeman D, Sheaves B, Goodwin GM, et al. The effects of improving sleep on mental health (OASIS): a randomised controlled trial with mediation analysis. Lancet Psychiatr 2017;4(10):749–58.

Printed and bound by CPI Group (UK) Ltd, Croydon, CR0 4YY

03/10/2024

01040367-0007